Adolescent Suicide

Adolescent Suicide

Formulated by the
Committee on Adolescence

Group for the Advancement of Psychiatry

Report No. 140

Published by

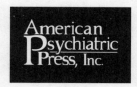

American
Psychiatric
Press, Inc.

Washington, DC
London, England

Copyright © 1996 Group for the Advancement of Psychiatry
ALL RIGHTS RESERVED
Manufactured in the United States of America on acid-free paper
99 98 97 96   4 3 2 1

Published by American Psychiatric Press, Inc.
1400 K Street, N.W., Washington, DC 20005

Library of Congress Cataloging-in-Publication Data
Adolescent suicide / formulated by the Committee on Adolescence.
        p.   cm. — (Report / Group for the Advancement of Psychiatry ;
     no. 140)
     Includes index.
     ISBN 0-87318-208-1
     1. Teenagers—Suicidal behavior.   2. Suicide—Prevention.
     3. Adolescent psychotherapy.   I. Group for the Advancement of
     Psychiatry.   Committee on Adolescence.   II. Series: Report (Group
     for the Advancement of Psychiatry : 1984) ; no. 140.
     RC321.G7   no. 140
     [RJ506.S9]
     616.89 s--dc20
     [616.85'8445'00835]   95-47286
                                                                            CIP

British Library Cataloguing in Publication Data
A CIP record is available from the British Library.

Contents

Introduction

This report has been formulated by a committee of child and adolescent psychiatrists who in clinical practice are engaged in relieving disease and disorder and furthering the strengths and development of their patients.

From its beginning, the committee has focused its attention on the adolescent process itself. Discussions have embraced the three determinants universal for all ages: biology, culture, and psychology. In its first report, *Normal Adolescence: Its Dynamics and Impact* (1968), the committee emphasized that adolescence is a constructive stage in human development, both for the adolescent and for society. The committee hoped that the presentation of the psychodynamics of normal adolescence would increase the understanding and rapport between the adolescent and adult generations.

In its second report, *Power and Authority in Adolescence: The Origins and Resolutions of Intergenerational Conflict* (1978), the committee elaborated the transition from the use of power and authority by adults to its acquisition by developing adolescents. The committee emphasized the importance of intergenerational communication and negotiation and considered structures that fostered and structures that inhibited successful adolescent development.

In its third report, *Teenage Pregnancy: Impact on Adolescent Development* (1986), the committee began its consideration of situations that threatened the adolescent process and therefore subsumed the report under the heading *Crises of Adolescence*. The committee noted that teenage pregnancy is not a single syndrome. Pregnancy in an adolescent need not have devastating results to the adolescent mother and father.

Some adolescents may turn the crisis into a growth-inducing experience. Nevertheless, as the report emphasized, unmarried teenage girls seldom become pregnant for sound reasons. Pregnancy and its consequences too often lead to an increased risk of social and psychological impoverishment, in great measure because of the disruptions of the development of the adolescent from childhood to adulthood. The report described methods of intervention by which clinicians may safeguard the development of the adolescent. The report considered prevention of pregnancy, abortion, carrying the pregnancy to term, delivery, giving up the infant for adoption, and keeping the baby and assuming the responsibilities of parenthood. The committee was concerned with the impact of teenage pregnancy on the development of the adolescent and on the development of the infant to be born. The committee recognized that teenage pregnancy represents a crisis in adolescence that may be disastrous but that may provide the adolescent with an opportunity to learn to cope with a stressful situation and possibly to create a hopeful future.

In this report regarding adolescent suicide, the committee addresses a crisis in the adolescent, in the extreme of which coping with stress is impossible. Suicidal adolescents can no longer bear their pain. They relinquish communication and negotiation with others. Their isolation is complete. They lose hope and abandon the future. Attempted suicide is not only a crisis in adolescent development, it is a crisis in adolescent existence. However, as in the case of teenage pregnancy, adolescent suicidal ideation, threats, gestures, attempts, and completion do not comprise a single syndrome or a series of syndromes. Except for completed suicides, they may provide a signal that communicates need and despair, a signal to which a responsive environment can rally to restore and further the process of health and adaptation. Thus, the risk of suicide presents an unparalleled crisis in adolescent development, a crisis that crystallizes our awareness of the impact of the biological and psychological thrusts of adolescence with the cultural and interpersonal tasks of society. For this reason, and because this life-threatening crisis can be clarified and hopefully modified through an understanding of the development of the adolescent, the committee has brought its perspective on adolescent development to the problem of adolescent suicide.

The committee is concerned as well about the meaning to society of the increasing incidence, for indeed it is increasing, of adolescent suicide. If, as we believe, adolescence is a constructive stage in human development, not only for the adolescent but for society as a whole, what does this increase in suicidal behavior reveal to us? What does it portend? What is our loss? Erik Erikson (1964) noted: "As cultures, through graded training, enter into the fiber of young individuals, they also absorb into their lifeblood the rejuvenative power of youth. Adolescence is thus a vital regenerator in the process of social evolution; for youth selectively offers its loyalties and energies to the conservation of that which feels true to them and to the correction or destruction of that which has lost its regenerative significance." That is our loss.

This report elucidates the biological, cultural, and psychological factors that influence the development of the adolescent within society. It will consider factors that have contributed to the breakdown of the full potential of the adolescent process with the destruction, through suicide, of the element of regenerative significance, the life of the adolescent. The report offers measures by which psychiatrists and all those caring for the health and welfare of adolescents can respond to their signals of distress with timely therapeutic intervention and suggests measures of anticipatory prevention.

An Illustrative Example

Even with careful assessment and competent psychiatric intervention, it is difficult, if not impossible, to predict the suicidality of an individual. Then, psychiatrists have to confront the death of someone they have tried to help. Suicide is a deeply painful experience for the surviving family, friends, and the therapists who ask whether they could have done more. Physicians are trained to work with dying patients and become familiar with death from incurable illness; however, they are less likely to accept as inevitable a patient's suicide. Yet there are some patients determined to die no matter what is done. Even the most skilled therapist may not know what action to take and may underestimate the suicide potential.

What follows is the presentation of a completed suicide. As such, it best illustrates many of the complex issues raised when working with these youngsters. Although it is a discouraging example, it illustrates some of the difficulties, risks, and crucial uncertainties facing the therapist who attempts to evaluate and then to initiate therapy with an adolescent whose history and early self-presentation provide no clear-cut indications of imminent suicidal risk.

Roger, an 18-year-old college student, asked for an evaluation several months after his 60-year-old father had phoned because he believed that

Roger was not doing well in his freshman year of college and had encouraged his son to return home and get involved in psychotherapy. He had been referred by his father's psychiatrist whom the father had been seeing in psychotherapy for many years. When Roger called, he said that he wanted therapy for reasons different from his father's.

In the office a few days later, Roger explained that his father was unnecessarily concerned about his alcohol use at college and his poor grades, but he was evasive about what his father meant. Roger had come home to live with his father and enrolled at a local college. What concerned the patient most is that he was fired from his job at a fast-food restaurant about a month before because he worked too slowly, was forgetful, and felt less competent than his co-workers. More recently, he had felt depressed and suicidal. He had no definite plan, nor had he felt a strong urge to kill himself. He said that his mother had died of cancer 7 years earlier when he was 11, cried about it in the initial session, and expressed surprise that her death still affected him so strongly. He said that he was now doing well in school and drinking less.

The initial impression was that Roger was experiencing unresolved grief over the death of his mother, was depressed, and might have significant problems with alcohol or substance abuse.

Three days later, Roger was puzzled by what psychotherapy is and how it would help him, especially because he would prefer to avoid painful discussions of his mother's death. He seemed blocked from memories of her. A 10-year-old sister had died from a brain tumor about 2 years before he was born, and he believed that this death had affected his older sister and his parents.

While he was away at school, he became more interested in his family's religion, an important part of his family's life up until his mother's death. Roger could remember no behavioral problems or symptoms in childhood, except for occasional fist fights. About 6 months before, he had a fight with a cousin who had accused him of being an alcoholic; this was the episode that had apparently prompted his father to insist he come home and get into therapy. Roger denied significant drug or alcohol usage. He was sexually active but often felt shy and "inadequate" with women. He said that the first session had increased his feelings of depression, and he seemed reluctant to leave the office.

In the third session, a week later, he acknowledged that he had thought of himself as a "replacement" for his deceased sister. One year after his sister's death, his mother overdosed, although this was never discussed in the family; Roger recognized a family tendency to avoid discussing painful issues. As a result of these three diagnostic interviews, the psychiatrist recommended psychotherapy and discussed with Roger the process and the frequency of sessions; Roger said that he would like to think it over.

One week later, in the office, Roger said that he had decided to schedule once-a-week sessions. He had been drinking at a fraternity party the night before, felt lonely, shy, "out of place," and friendless and had some transient suicidal thoughts. Before the next session, he called twice and seemed to be grieving, sporadically. In the next session, a Thursday, he reported that he would often cry with no images but other times had memories of his mother. At times, he felt choked up and found it hard to breathe and was talking a lot with friends about his mother. He asked for twice-a-week sessions, and Mondays and Thursdays were scheduled.

The following Monday, he said that he was no longer feeling so moved by the loss of his mother and even wondered if he had been forcing it. As he was about to leave the session, he said that he would no longer need to come in twice a week and wanted to cut back to once a week. The psychiatrist refused to do this and said they needed to discuss this further on Thursday. Roger seemed to agree but called that Monday evening to say that he insisted on cutting back to once a week, that he was canceling the next two sessions, Thursday and Monday, and would be in Thursday of the following week. The psychiatrist disagreed with him, told him they needed to talk this over but continue with the schedule as planned, and emphasized how important it was he keep these appointments.

Roger's father phoned about 11:30 P.M. the next day, Tuesday, to say Roger had killed himself by jumping off the roof of the parking garage next to the therapist's office building at about 3:00 P.M. while the psychiatrist was in his office. He died a few hours later at a local hospital.

His father said that Roger had been doing better and had been pleased with an A in a course and that he knew Roger had wanted to cancel the sessions and that the psychiatrist had refused. He expressed shock and surprise at Roger's suicide and said Sunday night Roger had been laughing when talking on the phone with a female friend. The note Roger left his father said that he loved him, that he hated to give his father another loss after the death of his sister and mother but that he could not go on and suicide was "inevitable," and that, since his mother died, he was depressed and there was no alternative. He thanked his father for trying to help him by getting him into therapy. He said he was going to jump off the building where his father had come looking for him the day before, something the therapist did not know. His father explained that, after Roger's Monday therapy session, he could not get his car started because he left the headlights on and the battery had run down. He called his father and asked him to come to the adjacent parking garage for a battery jump. By the time his father arrived, Roger had been helped by a security guard and gone home.

Roger had discussed his suicidal ideation, and the psychiatrist did not think he was at immediate risk because he had no plan, no lethality,

no strong urges. However, there was a family history of a suicide attempt, a family history of depression, a death he experienced, and another in the family as well. Other important factors are that he was male,
he used alcohol, and he was impulsive. His history did not substantiate
a career of impulsivity, except for the fight with his cousin and his behavior in suddenly deciding to decrease the frequency of the sessions.
Some depressed individuals feel better when they have decided on suicide and have a plan, but Roger had said that he would keep his Thursday appointment the following week.

Roger's jump from the adjacent building relates the suicide to the
therapeutic relationship. He wrote his father an explicit note, maybe
hoping he would stop him, but his father was at work. Roger may have
come by the office to see the psychiatrist, but there is no way of knowing. He may have been enraged with his therapist. No evidence exists of
a psychotic transference or a strong or irreversible regression, and he
seemed to be developing an alliance in the first six sessions. The therapist recognized that Roger was grieving and that this had been mobilized by interpreting the significance of his mother's death to him. The
psychiatrist believed he was in empathic contact with Roger.

In retrospect, Roger had several suicide risk factors:

- The death of his mother with unresolved grief;
- Clinical depression with a drop in academic and work performance,
  poor concentration, low self-esteem, and suicidal ideation;
- Alcohol abuse;
- Family history of depression and suicide attempt;
- Impulsivity; and
- Denial as a chief defense mechanism.

The psychiatrist might have interviewed the father to obtain more information. Could this suicide have been prevented? Every clinician must
ask this question, even though there will be instances when valid prediction is impossible even with additional historical information and in
which nothing or no one could have prevented the suicide.

This report explores these and other risk factors, the identification
and evaluation of the suicidal adolescent, and approaches to therapy. It
also presents a historical and cross-cultural perspective, the relevance
of suicide to adolescent development, mental health training needs regarding suicidality, and related issues such as public health policies and
medicolegal concerns.

Suicide in Historical, Cross-Cultural, and Sociological Perspectives

Voluntary self-destruction seems so totally contrary to any logical concept of natural selection that it is difficult to rationalize a place for it from an evolutionary perspective (de Catanzano 1981; D. H. Rubinstein 1986). It appears not to exist naturally, to any appreciable degree, among nonhuman animals. Such seemingly suicidal behavior as that of Norwegian lemmings actually occurs by accident during the course of adaptive behavior: migration away from an area of depleted food supply and over-population. Among humans, however, it is too widespread to dismiss as an exotic rarity.

Altruistic suicide—the voluntary death of one or more individuals for the good of the group—is evolutionarily reasonable from a sociobiological point of view, but this accounts for but a small minority of suicides. Analogous behavior among nonreproducing members of symbiotic colonies of social insects does occur (e.g., worker honey bees and soldier castes of various species of termites and ants), but it would be anthropomorphizing to impute a conscious motive. It is possible that because the majority of humans live in conditions that are far removed from their environment of evolutionary adaptedness, these rapid (in evolutionary terms) cultural and environmental changes constitute a chronic disorganizing stress. Self-damaging behavior does occur among other species in the unnatural environments of captivity and cages, but suicide among Stone Age peoples presumably living in environments more analogous to that of hominid evolution argues that this explanation of suicide is not an inclusive one. Chronic stress can deplete central nervous system neurotransmitters such as serotonin and norepinephrine, and there is research evidence linking such depletion to suicide even in the absence of diagnosed depression. Cognitive and behavioral flexibility has unquestionable natural selection advantages, and this basically adaptive development may carry the built-in risk that such flexibility can misfire in maladaptive ways. The fact that suicide is primarily or solely a human behavior points to the crucial importance of a high degree of cognition and learning and consequent cultural development and differentiation. Broad concepts of how it is possible for the species to evolve nonsurvival behaviors, however, do not, except in altruistic suicides, get one much further in understanding why most individuals tolerate the current evolutionary status of the species, whereas others do not, nor do they provide adequate explanation for the wide variation in suicide incidence in different cultures.

The focus of this book is suicide in adolescence. There are few cross-cultural data that focus on adolescence or distinguish suicide in that developmental stage from suicide in other life stages. Despite the recent surge of interest in adolescent suicide in Western culture, the data are more demographically comparative than culturally and developmentally descriptive. Even in the literature that purports to consider adolescent suicide specifically, youth up to, or even averaging, age 25 often are lumped with those in the teens in the same statistical or conceptual category. In addition, the bulk of the material that does address adolescent suicide is more cross-national within Western culture than truly cross-cultural, although Japanese and Amerindian cultures are notable exceptions.

The cross-cultural suicide studies that do exist are not irrelevant or inapplicable, however, even when they do not separate out adolescence. The same aspects of cultural differences that bear on the unique suicidality of a particular culture also impinge on its adolescents. In this chapter, we present a brief overview and synthesis of historical and cross-cultural perspectives on suicide and then look at what may be specific to adolescence and in what ways the developmental dynamics of adolescence give a special cast to the cultural differences.

Historical Aspects of Suicide

The "history" of suicide is culture specific; each culture has its own past and evolving patterns of and attitudes toward suicide. Regardless of the culture, however, two threads of suicidal meaning can be traced throughout its sociocultural history: social or institutional suicide and individual or personal suicide (Farberow 1975). In the first, society demands suicide as part of the individual's identification with the group and prescribes or approves the appropriate occasions for suicide, and often the form as well. Examples are sacrificing one's life for one's country, dying with one's king, or removing oneself in age or sickness as a burden to one's family or clan. In the second, suicide is a protest against personal pain or despair. Examples are suicide to escape dishonor or slavery, despair over rejection by or the loss of a love object, or escape from intolerable oppression or physical illness and pain.

It is not possible directly to trace historical aspects of suicide in the preliterate periods of human development or in existing preliterate peoples. The earlier anthropological view that suicide was rare or absent among primitive peoples has not held up in more careful ethnographic data (see de Catanzano 1981, for references and a brief review of data). Suicide is reported in almost all cultures specifically studied for it, although the rates vary across preliterate cultures as widely as they do among literate and industrialized cultures. Suicide is generally considered to be extremely rare among Australian aborigines, for example, whereas it reaches a rate of 53 to 70 per 100,000 in one Polynesian group (*Tikopia*)—several times higher than in any industrialized culture (de Catanzano 1981). As in the Western world, suicide rates are typically higher in men than in women in primitive cultures, but here, too, there are exceptions. Among the Muria of India the gender ratio is equal, and more women than men kill themselves among the Soga of Uganda. Both institutional and personal suicides occur among primitive groups, the relative incidence depending on cultural values, although some instances of both types are usually reported. Altruistic suicides among elderly and infirm persons were common among many Eskimo groups in precontact times, and suicide for personal reasons was reportedly common among the Trobrianders. Hanging is by far the most common means of suicide among primitive peoples, but again this is not without exception.

By definition, reports of suicide in the preliterate are produced by literate outsiders, after there has been contact with and intervention by more developed cultures. Such reports, nevertheless, cannot be discounted as simply reflecting intervention and acculturation stress. Many of the studies derive from earliest contact and describe native accounts of precontact conditions. Methods are also often specific to the native culture and different from those of the contact peoples, and some studies found suicide more prevalent in those areas of a culture with the least contact with the more advanced outsiders.

In Japan, suicide has traditionally been not only sanctioned, but glorified (DeVos 1968; Jilek-Aall 1988). Whether ritually prescribed, as in the hara-kiri of the Samurai class and similarly motivated individuals in recent times, or personally motivated, such as suicides of romantically frustrated or despairing individuals, suicide is an honorable resolution of unsolvable dilemmas. The tremendous traditional responsibilities of the individual to family and cultural expectations weigh about as heavily on both genders, although in different ways. In part because suicide is a culturally accepted way out, the overall suicide rates are relatively high when compared with other industrialized cultures or countries. The sex ratio is almost equal, the suicide rate for females being the highest among modern nations. Data regarding China are less readily available, but what exists indicate very similar cultural attitudes toward suicide.

The Brahmins of India regarded suicide favorably as an admirable manner of turning away from the world and gaining access to the spiritual plane. Suttee, in which a widow would be cremated on the funeral pyre of her husband, was common until very recently and was practiced in many parts of the orient. Throughout the Orient, suicide was common and generally accepted or honored. In contemporary India, suicide rates are lower overall than in Western cultures, but they vary enormously depending on local ethnic differences, and the gender ratios of suicides by men and women are equal. A significant difference in comparison with the West is that suicide is higher among married women than among single and divorced women. It is suggested (Adityanjee 1986) that this is caused in part by problems relating to dowries and to the mistreatment of the subservient wives in the extended families of the husband.

Attitudes toward and practices of suicide in Judeo-Christian (including the Graeco-Roman) culture have changed many times (Choron 1972; Farberow 1975). The Greeks of Homeric times regarded suicide as natural and appropriate in a variety of life circumstances that they considered untenable, such as after the commission of a horrible crime, conditions of dishonor, unrequited love or loss of love, and as acts of heroism for country or for another person. In post-Homeric times there arose a great pessimism about the value and condition of life, and many philosophers and groups openly encouraged suicide simply as a means of ending the misery of being alive and having to witness and endure the depravity and cruelty of the period. Attitudes and suicidal behaviors in the Roman Republic were essentially the same as among the Greeks. In the Roman Empire, the government officially disapproved of suicide, but in practice there was a generally permissive attitude toward it except when the interests of the state or of property were involved. Disillusionment and pessimism about life affected Roman philosophy and thought as well; personal afflictions of all sorts and boredom and purposelessness were considered adequate justification for suicide. In Choron's historical review it is mentioned that the municipal senate of Marseilles supplied free hemlock to anyone with a valid reason for suicide.

Suicide was apparently uncommon among the ancient Hebrews; it remains so in Israel today. Because of the Hebrews' valuation of life and of God's wisdom, suicides were considered deranged and were therefore not culturally condemned. There is no condemnation of suicide in either the Old or the New Testament, and early Christianity did not particularly oppose it. Suicide was frequent among early Christians to escape persecution and became popular as a way to gain heaven quickly. Perhaps in part because of the latter reason, there was growing opposition by the church, a position that was stated in terms of categorical rejection and sinfulness by St. Augustine by the end of the 4th century A.D. This position was unequivocal throughout the Middle Ages, although suicides continued to occur among persecuted minorities, among non-Christians who refused to convert, and among people in general who were unwilling to endure, or were terrified by, the grinding realities of life and illness (such as the plague) in those times.

The Renaissance brought about the recrudescence of the philosophy of humankind as shaper of its own destiny and of the individual as master of his or her own fate. Suicide found many apologists among the philosophers of the day, such as Erasmus and Robert Burton; some were even in the church, as were Sir Thomas More and John Donne. This trend continued in such writers as Rousseau and David Hume. The principal philosophic opposition to the freedom of suicide came, as it always has and continues through the present, from all the major religions that influence and are part of Judeo-Christian culture. Islam, although not technically subsumed within Judeo-Christianity, has always completely and severely condemned suicide. Judaism also came to reject it but does its best to find reasons to excuse it in Jews who do kill themselves (Grolman 1988). Both Catholicism and Protestantism have never deviated from the position that suicide is a sin, although some of their more humanist theologians have proposed more moderate attitudes.

Farberow (1975) has suggested that the changes in the acceptance or condemnation of suicide over the history of Judeo-Christian culture have reflected shifting periods of authoritarian rejection of individualism and the right to individual reason versus periods of respect for the individual and of the right to reason and to question dogma. In primitive societies, attitudes toward death and suicide were governed primarily by magical thinking and superstitious ideas about and fears of the dead and their spirits. These ideas found their way into emerging religions and, Farberow considers, became the basis for the condemnation and "sinfulness" of suicide. The Greeks and the Romans largely respected individualism and reason, and tended to regard suicide as an individual right. As Christianity and later Muhammadanism became increasingly influential, their authoritarian nature denied the individual right to question dogma, and because suicide was condemned, it could not be regarded as an individual choice. The rise of individualism and reason in the Renaissance brought back the concept of reasonable suicide by individual choice, and the debate between religious authority and individual reason and control of one's destiny continues to the present. Throughout most of history, suicide was a moral, philosophical, or political issue. It was not until the 19th century that interest shifted from viewing suicide from those perspectives to viewing it predominantly in terms of its causes.

Mass or cluster suicides also have a long and worldwide history. In A.D. 74, some 960 Jews are reported to have killed themselves at Masada to avoid capture, execution, rape, and enslavement by the Romans. There were other mass suicides of Jews in the Middle Ages to avoid oppression and torture. Still other mass suicides of Jews and other non-Christians occurred to avoid enforced conversion. Mass suicide among persecuted heretical sects of Christians, such as the Albigensians in 13th century France, were frequent. As late as the 17th century, Russian schismatics preferred mass suicide to the enforced reforms of the Russian Orthodox Church. In this century, there are records of hundreds of people in Japan committing suicide by imitation or contagion following glorified incidents of individual, romantically inspired suicides. Cluster suicides continue today among adolescents (see p. 17).

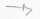 ## Sociological Perspectives on Suicide

Sociology studies the external social forces as causes of or reasons for behavioral differences in groups of people. Most contemporary sociologists recognize that valid explanations also entail interpersonal and intrapsychic causation and that pure sociology is a simplistic approach to human behavior. It is useful, though, to explore the understandings of suicide attributed to social forces in this section and to look at the contributions of psychodynamics (as they express themselves individually, interpersonally, and culturally) in the next section. It will be seen, however, that the distinction is so artificial that some consideration of psychological factors enters into many sociological approaches as well (see Choron 1972 and Group for the Advancement of Psychiatry 1989). Durkheim (1951) was the first to attempt a cohesive categorization of the social causes of suicide that could apply cross-culturally. He viewed society as a system that constrained and regulated the individual's behavior by means of societal integration and regulation, and he regarded suicide as generally contrary to societal well-being. Integration was defined in terms of the society's efforts and success in bringing its individual members to subordinate their individual interests in favor of such socially positive qualities and endeavors as ties to religion, family, and politics. Regulation was defined as the legitimate economic or domestic discipline or control that the society could exert over the individual. In Durkheim's study of the then available cross-cultural suicide statistics, degrees of social integration and regulation determined not only the different incidences but also different basic types of suicide. In general, cultures with very high or very low rates of integration or regulation had higher suicide rates than did those that were moderately integrated or regulated. Egoistic and altruistic suicide occur at opposite extremes of the dimension of societal integration. At one extreme, egoistic suicide is defined as that which results from excessive individualism, in which individuals are inadequately bound to and integrated into the overall social good and may then commit suicide for personal reasons regardless of its effect on the social fabric. At the other extreme, altruistic suicide results from an exaggerated concern for the community and an excessive sense of duty. (It is difficult, even in Durkheim's perspective, to understand how this motivation for suicide harms society unless it became a majority phenomenon.) Anomic and fatalistic suicide occur at opposite extremes of societal regulation. Anomic suicide is defined as that which occurs in inadequately organized and regulated societies; individuals kill themselves because the society provides insufficient social goals and pursuits around which to organize a sense of the meaning of life. Fatalistic suicide is a form of giving up; it occurs in overregulated societies in which it appears to some individuals that personal gratifications and reasons to remain alive are overwhelmed by societal controls.

Subsequent studies have modified, expanded, and even negated Durkheim's theories as better statistics and as more inclusive and incisive concepts have been proposed, but they remain the benchmark against which other sociological theories are compared. Subsequent theories have more clearly included psychological variables. Social frustration, the degree to which an individual feels the master of his or her fate, was postulated to predispose toward suicide in the upper classes because they can less easily blame others for their distresses (Henry and Short 1954, 1957). However, studies by McGuinies et al. (1974) and Boor (1976) found a higher suicide rate in cultures that foster a high perception of an external locus of control than in those fostering a sense of internal locus of control, the former possibly related to a sense of helplessness. Jeffries (1952) added "Samsonic" suicide to Durkheim's basic types. In this type of suicide, the culturally perceived motivation is to exert a vengeful, punitive, or even corrective effect on the offending survivors or on the culture itself. A common form of this in a wide variety of preliterate cultures is the suicide of a woman excessively abused according to cultural norms; her death predictably brings vengeance by her support group of kin on the offender, usually her husband. This motivation is clear in the case of the Japanese emperor's emissary who was sent to Manchuria at the end of World War II to instruct the forces there to surrender. When the officers refused, the emissary returned to his plane and had it crashed directly in front of them, killing himself and all aboard. This dramatic action forced the officers to obey and surrender (described in a different context in DeVos 1968).

Masamura (1977) directly tested Durkheim's hypotheses in a broad worldwide cross-cultural sample and found the suicide rate the opposite of that proposed by Durkheim; the more highly integrated the overall society, the higher the suicide rate. He postulated that suicidality is related to individual rather than social integration, in that an isolated or alienated individual in a highly integrated society would feel more isolated than one in a loosely integrated society; he or she would therefore be more likely to be ostracized, have little support, feel more different from others, and commit suicide more readily.

On the other hand, D. H. Smith and Hackathorn (1982) studied the World Ethnographic Sample in the Human Relations Area Files and found that suicide is lowest in cultures in which there is greater family, political, and economic integration; the latter refers to nomadic or seminomadic groups with a small local community size and a hunter-gatherer economy and in which individuals are highly interdependent. Other determinants of a low suicide rate found in this study were a moderate emotional expressiveness (versus very self-contained or highly expressive) and a low cultural focus on pride and shame.

Some studies have addressed the changing status of women as an influence on suicide rates. Stack (1978) found that the highest correlation with increased suicide rates in industrialized nations was the degree of female integration into the labor force. This integration correlated with higher female suicide rates, but parallel male rates increased even more sharply. He postulated that this change in female role and status may set off feelings of inadequacy and failure in men. Vigderhous and Fishman (1977) found that the most important variable with respect to female suicide was not work-force participation per se, but the effect of the female's occupation on family integration. Where the woman's occupation correlates with family dissolution or small family size, there is a higher female suicide rate.

Acculturation stresses constitute a special but enormously important consideration in regard to suicide in a world in which relatively few cultures remain isolated from outside influence and smaller, less technologically advanced cultures stand little chance of surviving against the onslaught of highly developed, expanding, and acquisitive cultures. Anthropological studies are unanimous in finding that the forced disruption of a culture results in increased suicide incidence within the original culture. This holds true regardless of how diverse the original culture may be (Kahn 1982) and often contradicts Durkheim's hypotheses. In comparing suicide rates among Navajo, Pueblo, and Apache Indians, it was found that although the Pueblo groups are more socially integrated than are the Navajo, their suicide rates are higher, and among the different Pueblos, suicide varied directly with the degree to which each was subjected to acculturation. The suicide rates in the three groups (highest for Apache and lowest for Navajo) reflected the degree to which there had been a forced change of culture (Van Winkle and May 1986).

Acculturation stress, however, is a concept too broad and undifferentiated to account for the great variation in how different cultures and individuals respond to such stress. Although Amerind suicide rates are alarmingly high following acculturation, Shore (1975) has shown that the rates of different groups vary greatly. Rates of some groups are much higher than the national average, whereas others (notably the Navajo) are no higher. The GAP Report (1989) on suicide and ethnicity in the United States proposes a sophisticated and interactive psychocultural model for understanding the varying outcomes of acculturation and their influence on suicidality. This model takes into account ". . . the phase of acculturation, the mode of acculturation, the type of acculturating group, the nature of the more dominant cultural group or society, the sociocultural characteristics of the less dominant group, and the psychological characteristics of the acculturating individuals." Such an approach goes a long way in facilitating an understanding of the variables that help

determine the despair or the resilience of cultures and individuals subjected to the stresses of cultural disruption.

Of all the efforts to integrate sociological concepts of suicide, that
by DeVos (1968) seems the most comprehensive. His is actually a totally
integrative approach, encompassing both social and psychological variables, but it is better considered as sociological in that it is less specific
about individual psychodynamics than about broad sociopsychological
variables. He ignores Durkheim's category of fatalistic suicide and adds
the category of acute interpersonal suicide. In a complex and inclusive
matrix of interacting social and individual psychological influences and
variables, DeVos provides a model that allows the exploration of the
social, interpersonal, and intrapsychic meanings and motivations of any
instance of suicide about which adequate information is available. Although his paper is densely written and sometimes difficult to understand, it does provide a genuinely comprehensive set of dimensions by
which to conceptualize suicide. His extensive discussion of various examples of suicide in Japan, according to his conceptual dimensions, provides an excellent example of the usefulness of his model.

Medical-psychiatric approaches to the understanding of suicide are
a special aspect of the sociological and psychological inquiries into causation. The relevance of mental states to suicide was assumed as far back
as Hippocrates, who noted that maidens "afflicted with menstrual problems and accompanying mental disorders were commonly suicidal" (de
Catanzano 1981, p. 26). Modern medical inquiries began perhaps with
Esquirol (1838/1965), who considered suicide a symptom of insanity,
and de Boismont (1865), who differentiated suicides in "reasonable
people" and in people who were insane. Freud sought throughout his
productive life to explain the intrapsychic motives of self-destruction.
Contemporary medical explanations fall into two broad, overlapping
categories of concepts. There are those that seek a psychogenic and
psychodynamic source for feelings of despair, desperation, self-directed
rage, helplessness, and hopelessness. There are explanations that focus
on diagnosable mental illnesses that imply genetic and biological eti-
ologies at least in significant part. However, it is clear that psychogenic
conditions associated with suicidal behavior are inevitably accompanied by neurobiological changes or conditions that are not characteristic
of the nonsuicidal mind.

No single explanatory concept of suicide is adequate in itself. The
purely sociological explanations offer no help in distinguishing between
those subject to a shared social condition who do commit suicide and
those who do not. Likewise, the medically extreme view that everyone

who commits suicide has a mental disorder is remarkably shortsighted in its failure to recognize many people in virtually all cultures who are subjected to such oppressively devastating and irremediable conditions of life that it would require some degree of mental disorder in such circumstances to be unaware of or to deny the extent of the hopelessness of life. Choron (1972, p. 4) noted that Ortega y Gasset (1932) "has pointed out, for most people at all times 'life' meant limitation, obligation, dependence, and oppression. They go on living simply because they happen to have been born, sustained by the force of habit, sometimes out of curiosity or vague hopes for a better future, and because they are afraid of the alternative—death."

Cross-Cultural Aspects of Suicide From the Perspective of Psychodynamics

The social conditions in different cultures that may have relevance to culturally differential suicidality are the outgrowth of beliefs, persistent magical thinking, attitudes, defenses, and preferred modes of coping that are shared by the members of the culture. These shared psychodynamics give rise to culture-specific institutions, including culture-specific childrearing philosophies and techniques, normative expectations of children and adults, and characteristic patterns of interpersonal relations and reactions to the perceived realities of life. To the extent that relatively uncontaminated cultures or groups are distinguishable from one another, their differences reflect different constellations of psychodynamic patterns. The cultural institutions that evolve from shared psychodynamics in turn operate to help determine culture-typical patterns of adaptive and maladaptive behavior in the individuals and group units of the culture. Suicide is one behavior that can be understood more clearly in the light of culturally shared psychodynamics.

A number of studies have focused on culturally characteristic childrearing patterns and their effects on adult ego development and defensive patterns. Hendin's (1978) study of Scandinavian suicide found that the high suicide rates in Sweden and Denmark and the low rate in Norway reflected differences in childrearing practices and the ego strengths, weaknesses, and typical defenses this fostered. In Denmark, there is great mother–child dependency and little encouragement of autonomy; the father is often distant and of little influence. Children are taught to restrain strong emotion, particularly anger, and they are imbued with a strong obligation to perform and succeed to gratify and reward their hard-working and self-sacrificing parent. They learn through maternal example that guilt is a very effective means of interpersonal control, and suicide is often openly intended to cause guilt in the survivors. Swedish children, especially males, are subject to early expectations of independence and performance in an atmosphere of relative maternal emotional detachment. The internalized demand for competitive success in the context of emotional flatness is correlated with a high rate of male suicide related to a sense of individual failure in persons with constricted emotional options for coping with personal disappointments. In Norway, there is little childrearing focus on competition and accomplishment in order to be accepted; children grow up to be less rigidly self-demanding. Parental roles are more traditionally patriarchal in Norwegian families, and there is less family dissolution than in Denmark; individualism, self-reliance, assertiveness, and cooperation over competition are fostered.

Jilek-Aall's (1988) cross-cultural study of suicide among youths confirms and extends Hendin's study and also includes data on Amerinds and Japanese. She points out other aspects of Danish and Norwegian childrearing and culture that correlate with their differential suicide rates. Norway is more sparsely populated; survival has always demanded family and community cooperation. Because of this caring interdependence in addition to their childrearing experiences, children have a more optimistic outlook, they believe there is always some way out of difficulties, and they can always count on a close kin and social network for support. Population density in Denmark is high, one's milieu consists largely of strangers, and there is little close, enduring social support network. There is one high-risk group in Norway: young men who have not been able to fit in with or accept traditional family and cultural values. They usually wind up as seamen, living in conditions that are totally different from the supportive aspects of traditional Norwegian culture.

In Japan, there is an extraordinary and extended physical and emotional closeness between mother and child that is almost symbiotic (see also DeVos 1968). The mother's life and hopes are largely lived through her children: for boys, educational and financial success; for girls, an appropriate and honorable marriage. The mother's goals are strongly internalized, and at the same time, emotional control and repression of anger are demanded. The cultural tradition inculcates great devotion to and respect for elders and for authority, and externalizing blame for any personal shortcomings onto outside circumstances or persons is discouraged. Because failings must be perceived as inner flaws, there is little psychocultural awareness of a need for external support systems for those in distress. There are few helping agencies for disturbed youths, and few seek help or communicate their suicidal thoughts. Suicide is a common response to the lonely sense of having failed to maintain one's family's (therefore one's own) sense of honor.

Jilek-Aall's material on Amerinds and Inuits primarily focuses on the postcontact and forced acculturation period. Here, the family disruption is externally caused, but the early childrearing deficits are seen as crucial in the failure of such youths to be able to provide themselves with the necessary emotional support of close friendships and one's own spouse and family or to be prepared to cope successfully with the realistically major task of succeeding in the real world of Western culture. In commenting on childrearing practices of the Mescalero Apache, Boyer (discussed in Hippler 1969) describes a pattern of rearing in which the infant is first adored and then emotionally abandoned (sometimes actually, through being given away) after the birth of the next child. The resulting pervasive hostility and deficits in the sense of self-worth and trust are acted out both aggressively and suicidally through what is called "suicidal drinking."

At the unconscious psychodynamic level, Hippler's (1969) analysis of cross-cultural suicidality offers a cogent synthesis of the influence of childrearing practices on cultural personality and institutions and the role of those institutions in reawakening characteristic forms and degrees of suicidal behavior in youths and adults. He points out that magical (primary process) thinking is universal, and all cultures institutionalize some aspects of it. Intrapsychic suicide motives are 1) fusion with an earlier, more gratified and peaceful state, the good mother, and 2) frustration of the expression of rage toward appropriate external objects so that it is vented against oneself, which is equivalent to injuring the frustrating party or the internalized bad parent. Often there are elements of both motives in the characteristic suicidal behavior of a particular culture. The wish for fusion is sometimes overt, as in expressions of a wish for reunion after death with mother or a maternal figure by some Danish suicides (Hendin 1978). When adult reality is irreconcilable with either real or retrospectively perceived infantile bliss, and childrearing did not foster more effective ways of coping with stress or of gaining realistic emotional support from others, magical fusion is a useful explanatory concept, for example, in some Japanese suicides. The vengeful or guilt-coercing motivation is often very clear, as in the self-poisoning of Iroquois women to bring social disapproval upon their husbands and in the Dobu man's suicide to provoke his lineage's revenge against an unfaithful wife.

Although examples such as these may seem to reflect specific cultural institutions rather than infantile psychodynamics and primary process thinking, social structures are not etiologically explanatory. Rather, they reflect shared psychodynamics and personality patterns and also serve to structure culturally typical interpersonal situations so as to elicit culturally suitable emotional expressions. Close attention to the childrearing practices and the accompanying expectations imposed on the children in a given culture reveals not only the degree to which unconscious wishes for fusion, or wishes to injure an internalized bad object, are fostered, but it also elucidates the manner in which those practices produce adults who create social structures and interpersonal situations, almost in the manner of self-fulfilling expectations, that reproduce the frustrations and conflicts of childhood. These structures and situations reelicit the person's unconscious motivations and create a scenario and cast of characters that provide for ready and obvious acting out of the unconscious wish with current substitute objects.

The degree to which magical thinking is institutionalized in a culture, and the constellation of ego strengths, weaknesses, and defenses produced by culture-specific childrearing practices, offer considerable insight into the etiology of cross-cultural differences in suicidality. Without such concepts, there can be no understanding of what created the specific institutions and cultural attitudes that seem to influence suicidal behavior so uniquely in diverse cultures.

The explanatory value of intrapsychic dynamics is not limited to the broad level of cultural differences, however. It is useful in comprehending some of the consequences of enforced cultural destruction and acculturation as they affect suicidality and in understanding individual instances of suicide. A common consequence of forced acculturation is the destruction of the traditional socioeconomic institutions that maintained the indigenous family structure and that both reflected and helped to structure childrearing practices. Families become disrupted in ways that no longer reflect stable precontact patterns. Financial hardship and parental maladaptive responses to loss of cultural identity result in children deprived of conditions necessary for the development of trust, a secure identity and self-worth, and the intrapsychic tools for successful adaptation. The real-life obstacles facing such children often leave few options other than magical escapes and regressions. When alcohol and other drugs are, or become, available, as with many Amerind groups, they are not only causes of suicidal acts, they are also symbolic, magical oral regressions to, and temporary (sometimes permanent) fusions with the real or fantasied and wished for good mother of infantile Nirvana. By releasing inhibitory controls, youths release the pent up aggressions, not only externally, but retroflexively toward the internalized bad parent. Traditional culture itself can come to represent the primordial good mother/good parent. Fusion with idealized ancestors is a conscious goal of some Amerind suicides. At the individual level, the unique early family milieu of any child in any culture may engender powerful unconscious needs for fusion or for self-directed aggression and produce such distorted capacity for interpersonal relationships that the person will unwittingly structure his or her personal social world to recreate and repeat the childhood traumas and trigger a maladaptive repair through suicide.

Adolescence as a Special Case

Ordinarily, adolescents would not be thought of as a group at high risk for suicide. Adults think of adolescents as being full of the excitement of life and its possibilities and of acceding to adult prerogatives. They are perceived as unacquainted yet with the full impact of the hardships and responsibilities of adulthood, and their cognitive immaturity prevents a full grasp of their individual limitations. That view, however, is both ethnocentric and uninformed about the circumstances of life for many adolescents. It is ethnocentric in that at its enlightened best, Western culture recognizes the importance of providing children with the best ego developmental and cognitive tools for rewarding adaptation in a difficult world. There are cultures in which that is a less thought-out goal, in which childrearing is psychologically crippling, and in which, by adolescence, hardships and limitations are all too obvious and adulthood is not a status that appears especially rewarding. It is uninformed in that even in Western culture, childrearing goals are often more honored in the breach than in the observance. Many families are socioeconomically incapable of providing the healthy emotional and educational building blocks for a successful adulthood. Many families that could provide them do not know how. Many ethnic and circumscribed socioeconomic groups in the West and elsewhere do not have adequate access to the social and financial resources that would make possible the healthy preparation of adolescents for adulthood. In addition, many cultures, including the Western cultures, are changing so rapidly that even those in the mainstream have lost the secure sense of a reasonably predictable life course for which to prepare children and adolescents.

In any of these less-than-optimal circumstances, the special characteristics of adolescence as an immature developmental stage place these

maybe

youngsters in an especially vulnerable position. At best, adolescents do
not yet have a secure sense of identity; they lack real accomplishment
and adaptive success in nondependent roles so as to have a valid self-
confidence. Because of their inner state of flux and unfinished personality development, they may have difficulty establishing firm and lasting
friendships and love relationships to sustain them through turmoil. Their
need to develop autonomy often distances them from parents and other
adult sources of emotional support.

The concept of autonomy deserves clarification. Although most ob-
servers of adolescents write about developing autonomy, they refer to a
psychological competence that often manifests itself in increasingly self-
reliant functioning. Most psychoanalytic and empirical studies of adolescent development do not demonstrate an internal detachment from
the important relationships of childhood—the parents—but rather a
transformation of those relationships and a shift in their intensity. Adolescents do not "separate" from their parents, but they do modify the
nature of that special attachment.

Thus, transformations occur in the nature of the adolescents' attachments and the attributes of those attachments. We infer that early omnipotence is resurgent in adolescence because the teenager is beset with
swings—from bravado to deflation, from blatant exhibitionism to shy-
ness, from hero worship to disparagement, from idealism to despair.
Early childhood grandiosity, already having undergone considerable
transformation in the preadolescent years, is now moved in the direction of establishing healthy self-esteem and reasonable ambitions. Early
idealization of omnipotent and omniscient parents shifts to establishing
one's own values and ideals and to respecting and admiring additional
adults. Adolescents do not simply use peers for sustaining relationships
in the way that they used to use parents for that purpose; rather, that
shift represents the development of increasing self-reliance. More and
more, the adolescent trusts his or her own capacities to regulate self-
esteem and enrich his or her purpose in life. Although this suggests a
marked movement toward autonomy, it does not mean that one detaches
from others, but simply uses them in different ways to sustain the self.

Their still immature level of ego development provides adolescents
with less stable defenses in the face of difficulties. This and the relatively recent transformations of puberty, which they have not yet fully
mastered, leave them prone to impulsivity. Magical thinking persists as
a developmental phenomenon, not only in those families and cultures
that foster it. In addition, both their own limitations and the perma-
nence of death are not sufficiently appreciated. When genuine depression

occurs in adolescence, it is often indirectly expressed, and that impairs recognition and help.

These developmental characteristics place adolescents at a heightened risk for inappropriate response to stress under the best of circumstances. Even a relatively minor perceived loss or rejection or disappointment in oneself can trigger self-destructive urges and behavior. When either the childrearing experiences or the cultural realities into which the adolescent is emerging compromise psychologically healthy development or realistically constrict the options for successful adult function, adolescents are particularly at risk for suicide.

This risk is clearly illustrated in cultures that figuratively tie many adolescents' adaptive hands. The suicidogenic nature of traditional Japanese childrearing and culture, where there has been one of the highest youth suicide rates among industrialized countries, has already been noted. Not only are the familial and cultural demands on young men often impossibly high, but the great competitiveness necessary for achievement and the limited mobility once an occupational choice is made effectively restrict the ability to achieve the aspirations that have been imposed (Li 1971). For women, arranged or at least parentally approved marriage is still common, and premarital chastity is expected. Young female suicide is especially high in Japan often as a result of unwed pregnancy or failure to obtain parental approval for a desired marriage (Jilek-Aall 1988). As traditional restraints break down under Westernization, Japanese youths are cast further adrift. The highly competitive demands for educational and financial success remain, but there are more actual or latent broken homes, and the adolescents are thrust into a peer world of premature sexual involvements and substance use (Kitamura 1983–85). This study found analogous conditions and high adolescent suicide rates in West Germany. Danish youths commit suicide two to four times more frequently than do Norwegian youths, correlated with differential cultural circumstances already described (Jilek-Aall 1988). Hendin (1978) has described culturally unresolvable conditions for black ghetto youths, in whom the suicide rate is very high. Theirs is a chronic exposure to violence and despair, both in everyday environment and often in families that are also bankrupt of financial and psychological resources to interpose against the external ghetto realities. These experiences engender more despair, rage, and murderous impulses, but the culture demands control of aggressive behavior; the aggression often erupts in self-directed as well as other-directed ways.

Cluster suicides among adolescents are especially difficult to comprehend on either a sociological or psychodynamic basis. Between one and two dozen clusters were reported between 1980 and 1987 in the United States, accounting for the deaths of at least 194 adolescents through age 20 (Coleman 1987). One fairly widely publicized cluster occurred in Plano, Texas, during a 15-month period. Eight adolescents committed suicide, beginning with that of a boy who had accidentally killed a close friend in an automobile accident. Seven boys and one girl committed suicide, and most knew each other and attended the same high school. Those who were not socially acquainted knew all about the others through intense media coverage. Four died from carbon monoxide poisoning (as had the first of the cluster), and four died of gunshot wounds. Three years after the first suicide, on the anniversary of that first death, a ninth boy committed suicide by the same means (Coleman 1987).

There has been considerable research into the meanings and mechanisms of suicide contagion and clusters; more questions than answers still exist. Imitation of and identification with the suicide victims are considered to be probable major factors, especially if the earlier victims are perceived to have had similar problems and distressing past experiences. Research clearly indicates that media coverage, particularly when it is extensive and in any way glamorizes the suicide, produces an increase of imitative suicides. There is a greater tendency toward an increase of suicides and suicide attempts if the original victims were in some way "attractive"—were celebrities or occupied high status. Social acquaintance with the other victims is a risk factor. It is possible that poor baseline emotional functioning increases susceptibility. Also, it may be that existing suicides in a community, and the attendant media coverage, may produce a familiarity with and an acceptance of suicide as a way out of difficulties, reducing the taboo or fear of suicide and lowering the threshold at which one may consider suicide as a potential solution for one's problems (L. Davidson and Gould 1989).

Adolescent suicide among Amerind and Inuit groups has received considerable study; it is highest in the 16- to 25-year-old group and also is very high for the 5- to 14-year-old group (Jilek-Aall 1988). Overall, the rate is 10 times higher than the national average (Davenport and Davenport 1987). The great variation in different tribes, however (Shore 1975), suggests that indigenous cultural and familial factors play a determinative role in adolescents' responses to the disintegration of their traditional cultures. The Navajo have a suicide rate same as the national average and have been notably successful maintaining traditional culture and values while accommodating to necessary acculturative changes. Eighty percent of Navajo suicides are in those who have forsaken traditional backgrounds (S. I. Miller and Shoenfield 1971).

Forced acculturation can be very hard on groups with a traditional ethos of internalizing emotions, such as the Arapaho and Shoshone tribes. Long (1986) reported an epidemic of nine suicides in youths between ages 14 and 26 years within 1 year in these tribes; all were known to each other. Ward and Fox (1977) also reported an epidemic of eight suicides, median age 22 years, in an unidentified tribe. All had been isolated since childhood, were generally noncommunicative, and had poor peer social skills; none had significant lovers or peer friends. They were therefore excessively dependent on parental families for their needs, yet all had experienced family discord, alcohol abuse, and loss and denigration by family members shortly before suicide. Their own main coping mechanisms had been withdrawal, internalization, and alcohol abuse; there had been many unheeded cries for help, and the eventual suicides were mostly planned rather than impulsive.

Dismang et al. (1974) also made a controlled study of suicides under age 25 years among the Shoshone, in which there is an unusually high suicide rate. Compared with nonsuicidal control subjects, all of the suicides had lost more than one significant caretaker before age 15, they had experienced two or more losses by desertion or divorce, their primary caretaker(s) had five or more arrests, and they were more likely to have attended boarding schools. The suicides and the control subjects all lived in the context of cultural disintegration, so the meanings of the suicides related more to familial and individual factors than to acculturative stresses. This conclusion is supported by a controlled study of suicide in Greenland (Grove and Lynge 1979). Most of the suicides were described as young, and the strongest correlation was with dysfunctional and alcoholic parental homes, rather than with broken homes per se, bereavement, or cross-cultural exposure. The suicides displayed alcoholism, criminality, and interpersonal conflicts.

It would appear that although there are broad cultural differences that correlate with differences in overall as well as adolescent suicidality, these differences are primarily useful at a potentially clinical level in calling attention to various areas of pathogenicity in childrearing and to unconstructive familial and cultural expectations that bear on adolescents in ways that conduce self-destructive behavior.

2

Normal Adolescent Development and Developmental Deviations: Relevance to Suicide

Psychological Factors in Adolescent Development

The definitions of puberty and adolescence are basic to the exploration of the relevance of adolescent development to adolescent suicide. Puberty is defined as the biological and physical changes that transform a child's body into that of an adult in size, function (including mental function), and procreative capacity. Adolescence is the psychosocial sequel to puberty. Adolescence is, by definition, an immature stage of human development. Although the biological changes in a healthy individual are pan-human, each child brings to that puberty, as tools to cope with its challenges and stresses, all the unique realities and influences that have gone before in his or her life, both good and bad.

The discussion that follows in this chapter applies primarily to developmental issues as they appear in youngsters in well-developed societies. Although there are issues in adolescence relating to the transformations of puberty and their consequences that transcend cultural differences, it cannot be assumed that this discussion applies with equal validity to cultures (e.g., Rwanda or Cambodia) vastly different from the highly developed technological cultures.

Most basic are that individual's particular genetic and constitutional characteristics, physical and anatomic realities such as size and vigor, and any past or present illness states that might affect the capacity to cope. The child's evolving intrapsychic self includes not only the sequelae of the normal and abnormal conflicts, transformations, and their resolutions from earlier developmental stages, but also innate areas of strength and vulnerability that reflect genetic and constitutional makeup. The effects of the child's particular childrearing and family relationships affect not only the intrapsychic self but also have begun to shape styles of interpersonal relatedness and patterns of interpersonal expectations. Added to this are the molding influences of all other important adults and peers. Finally, the culture and subculture or special ethnic group of which the child is part has had some overarching control over the family's approach to the child, the alternatives available, the flexibility with which the child is able to address the tasks of adolescence, and the adult world realities that will have to be faced.

Furthermore, adolescent development does not entail only the use of a child's preexisting tools; it takes place in the here-and-now real world in which the adolescent lives. The current realities of the youngster may differ in determinative ways from those of earlier life, such that they may make up for previous deficits or traumata, or undermine earlier and nascent strengths. Certain aspects of development can only occur after puberty and during adolescence, either because of an innate biological timetable or because they depend on the transformations of puberty as releasers of the opportunities to explore and integrate the new physical and psychological capacities. Psychological development unique to adolescence comprises many aspects of identity, of cognitive and moral development, of interpersonal style and relatedness, and of sexual and narcissistic changes.

Thus every puberty happens to a different person developmentally, and every adolescence reflects each youngster's currently unique biopsychosocial milieu. This does not mean, however, that adolescent development is random. The fact that *Homo sapiens* is a single species dictates some broad similarities. Within the wide gamut of differences, areas of commonality and even some degree of predictability may be discernible, to the degree to which one can become aware of the specific nature of the forces and influences that act on an adolescent's development.

Even in instances of sound innate biology and physical health, and in conditions that foster a youngster's potential for mastering the tasks of adolescence, there are characteristics inherent in adolescence as a developmental stage that may place adolescents at particular risk for suicide. Adolescence is an immature developmental stage, and that immaturity can confer a certain protection of innocence against some of the harsher future and even current realities. At the same time, adolescents have fewer psychological tools with which to manipulate the problems and stresses that arise.

Intrapsychic Aspects of Development

The cognitive capacity for what Piaget termed *formal operations* or propositional thought begins to be possible at about age 11 but probably is not fully capable of realization until about ages 14 to 16 (Inhelder and Piaget 1958). The younger child functions at the level of concrete operations, in which his or her thinking is limited by objects and operations that have been part of direct personal experience, and the range of his or her conceptual capacities is limited to the mental manipulation of concretely experienced objects. In formal operational thought, one is capable of thinking about propositions and possibilities one has never experienced. One is liberated from concrete experience and can imagine or fantasize the future consequences of different ideas and attitudes and courses of action without having to live them out and experience them in concrete reality.

In the healthy development of propositional thought, there is a normal function of suicidal fantasy for the adolescent. It is one aspect of the adolescent's coming to grips with the now (potentially) fully conceivable realities of life and death, mortality and immortality. There is a sense of power in the realization that "I can do something about my life if it becomes intolerable." In addition, fantasy can be an adaptive means of handling aggressive impulses, in this instance toward oneself; fantasy can decrease the need to act out in reality.

Age, however, is a necessary but insufficient criterion for achieving propositional thought. Once the brain matures sufficiently to make it possible, propositional thought must be fostered, valued, and taught by both the culture and the child's family or it will not develop. Even in the United States, where this level of cognition is generally valued and even crucial for effective function, almost 50% of all adolescents cannot pass the Piagetian tests that reveal formal operational thought (Kohlberg and Gilligan 1971).

Inadequate acquisition of propositional thought can impair the ability to see beyond a present loss or problem to a different and possibly better future. It can interfere with the ability to imagine how to accomplish a successful future based on appropriate preparation for it in the present. A cognitive incapacity to anticipate the future consequences of behavior without having had to experience them plays a major role in adolescent unplanned and unwed pregnancy. The crippling of one's sense of this inner capacity to influence one's destiny can lead to an assumption of an external locus of control of one's life and future, with the attendant sense of hopelessness and helplessness. These immature states of cognition can lead not only to literal suicide, but also to such forms of psychosocial suicide as substance abuse and antisocial behavior. On the other hand, Borst et al. (1991) have found that less advanced or delayed ego development can sometimes function as a protective factor against suicide, in that the youngster externalizes problems as being someone else's fault, rather than turning the aggression against the self.

The capacity for propositional thought, however, does not obviate adolescent despair. The adolescent who commits suicide in the face of some major dilemma or disaster (a diagnosis of AIDS, for example) that he or she realistically recognizes as severely compromising the future may be thinking more clearly than the adolescent who retreats into a drug-induced oblivion.

Even on a general level, the adolescent with greater cognitive capacity is not immune to suicidality. It is possible that the capacity for introspection increases suicidal risk and may even bring about the developmental emergence of suicide as a phase-specific behavior in adolescence. There is evidence that ego development enables the maturing personality to internalize emotional states and to experience more self-blame; this increases suicidal risk (Borst et al. 1991). The adolescent who displays a more internally structured personality, who relies less on contact with others for psychological self-support, may be less suicidal only because he or she is less prone to be impulsive and is more likely to delay gratification. However, the more structuralized youngster may be severely depressed and at great risk, especially because of the greater capacity for guilt and self-blame and because he or she has no capacity to use important others to console himself or herself.

Another normal characteristic of adolescent cognition is the persistence of magical thinking and primitive grandiosity. Along with even high intelligence and sophisticated cognition is the continuing sense that one is somehow immune to real consequences. It is doubtful that most adolescents who die as a result of Russian roulette took the likelihood of their death seriously. Even death is somehow magically not real and permanent. An extraordinarily bright 15-year-old girl once told one of the authors, "I really came very close to killing myself last night, but I knew that by today, I'd regret it."

The development of moral or principled thought follows an invariable sequence of stages that begin in earliest childhood, but the capacity for "postconventional" principles ("autonomous moral principles which have validity and application apart from the authority of the groups or persons who hold them and apart from the individual's identification with those persons or groups" [Kohlberg and Gilligan 1971, p. 1067]) is not possible until adolescence. Earlier stages of moral development entail behavioral self-control on the basis of punishment and reward and of the duty to follow rules to be liked and to support social order. Postconventional principled thought requires the capacity for propositional thought. However, just as the central nervous system capacity for formal operations did not ensure its achievement, the same is true here: Although approximately 60% of persons in their study over age 16 displayed propositional thought, only 10% showed postconventional principled thinking.

The relationship of this developmental line to adolescent suicide is subtle. The achievement of principled thought allows the adolescent to bring a less egocentric cognition to bear on personal problems and dilemmas, and much of adolescent suicide has an intensely egocentric cast.

The level of moral thought can vary in the same adolescent. In a study of the quality of moral thought that adolescents bring to the resolution of sexual versus nonsexual dilemmas, it was found that earlier, more primitive levels of moral thought were used in dealing with sexual problem solving (Gilligan et al. 1971). This less mature sexual decision making can lead to more damaging sexual behavior, the consequences of which place greater strain on an adolescent's coping skills. Problems in sexual relationships are a major risk factor in adolescent suicide.

Kohlberg's work and his conclusions grew from the use of male subjects. More recently, Gilligan (1982) studied the same developmental line in female subjects and found significant difference between the sexes. In the original description of postconventional thought, even at that level of moral thinking, the males revealed an individualistic approach that tended more rigidly to respect abstract principles and to take social relationships less into account. At the comparable level of moral development, females' solutions to moral dilemmas were more contingent, less dogmatic, and tended to place greatest emphasis on how decisions and solutions took into account and affected the relationships between people. By implication, even high-functioning males appear more isolated and inflexible in approaching moral dilemmas, of which suicide is certainly one. One may wonder whether there is some correlation between females' greater relatedness and the generally lesser rate of adolescent female suicide.

Identity development in adolescence is a broad and complex concept and is clearly influenced by the cognitive issues already discussed. This developmental task normally requires an extended period of modifying one's relationship with, often involving distancing oneself from, parents and usually other adults as well. This can deprive the adolescent of a vital sense of parental or adult emotional support at times of crisis. An adolescent may distance in a crude and hurtful way and may alienate parents in the process. These normal shifts away from parents, even without adversarial complications, are losses even while the adolescents are rebelling against the parents. These normal and healthy aspects of development have a side effect of isolation and depression, and such dynamics are often found to be precursors of attempted and completed suicide.

Because identity formation (and real world function consonant with that identity) is still in process, a secure knowledge of one's future self does not yet exist. A confident sense of one's probable future cannot be held onto as support through difficulties. The work of childhood and adolescence (measurable by the adult world) is school achievement and learning. For many adolescents, this is the only valid source of accomplishment to hold on to in times of stress, although popularity and athletic achievement can also serve as anchors of identity. Often this achievement does not confer the same degree of self-confidence and security that can be taken from more tangible, adultlike evidences of having succeeded in the real world. Furthermore, many of those who are not successful academically are fully capable of effective function in the predominately nonacademic sectors of the adult world. However, in the face of perceived losses or disasters, both those who are good and those who are not good at the work of school have relatively little tested and proven evidence of their capacity to sustain and overcome such traumata.

In Eriksonian terms (1968), adolescence is time of crisis and for consolidation of a psychosocial sense of identity; the failure of identity consolidation results in identity diffusion. The adolescent questions and reevaluates parental attitudes and values, and those of cultural institutions, in the process of arriving at a sense of self-in-the-world that is truly his or her own. This quality of questioning is prerequisite to the achievement of postconventional principled thought (M. H. Podd 1969, unpublished observations, cited in Kohlberg and Gilligan 1971). Identity foreclosure, the avoidance of the crisis of questioning, leaves the adolescent at the level of conventional morality, and the inability to resolve the process of identity formation resulting in identity diffusion leads to the inability to commit to any cohesive sense of self.

Identity diffusion clearly leaves the adolescent bereft of solid inner supports in the face of perceived severe stress. However, even in the potentially healthiest course of adolescent identity formation, that of going through the process of identity crisis, the adolescent is at risk of feeling psychologically adrift and therefore vulnerable to despair. In the course of this (usually temporary) repudiation of previously learned values and belief systems, there is little to which to anchor oneself. Repudiation creates a significant loss, however time-limited.

Sexual identity is a preeminent aspect of adolescent development, although it is not solely an adolescent phenomenon. Sexual differentiation begins in the fetal hormonal environment, and its most basic intrapsychic components are generally fixed by early childhood. It is in adolescence, however, that sexual development and sexual identity come to fruition, in the sense of being put to the test and being acted out, in the evolution of genitally mature sexual relationships.

At the intrapsychic level, innate male–female differences may play a role in the sex-differential adolescent suicide rates. There is convincing evidence that masculine identity is more difficult to achieve and more vulnerable to disruption than is feminine identity (Gadpaille 1972). Adolescent boys are hence more likely to be thrown into devastating self-doubt by the inevitable sociosexual losses and failures of adolescence than are girls. A sense of and a striving for bonding and relatedness are more basic to female than to male psychology. In the genetic consequences of evolution, a sense of mother-offspring bonding is earlier and more fundamental in female development than is either father-offspring or male-female bonding in the male (Gadpaille 1980, 1983). The intrapsychic consequence of the experience of early bonding for children of both sexes is to enable girl children to retain their primordial bond to mother without risk to their female identity, whereas boy children cannot do so (Gilligan 1982; Greenson 1968; Stoller 1974). Thus, females more than males potentially have a more innate and abiding sense of belongingness, with consequently less sense of isolation.

Throughout childhood, it is available, reliable, and consistent parental responsiveness that permits the developing child to modify his or her early grandiosity in the direction of mature self-esteem and realistic ambition. Such transformations begin before adolescence. The problems, arrests, and distortions of the preadolescent period influence the further modifications of adolescence. The idealization of parents by the adolescent begins to be modified in the direction of the adolescent's goals and values and of respect and admiration for others. The maturing adolescent can tolerate many inevitable painful experiences in the context of an emotionally sustaining milieu. The adolescent does not face tasks alone, even the task of modifying the emotional attachment to parents. Parents continue to sustain or fail the adolescent as before (Marohn 1980).

Adolescence is characterized by the resurgence of primitive self-regard with its associated problems. Adolescents may be brash and grandiose, or intimidated and self-depreciating. They may be preoccupied with the beauty or ugliness of their bodies, with their power and grace, or their weakness and clumsiness. They aggrandize themselves, or hate themselves. They may desperately seek others to sustain them and to reassure them, or isolate themselves, or change friends impetuously. They may be capricious in their crushes, their friendships, their feelings about parents, and their wanting to be alone. They may worship others as they once did their parents but may rapidly view today's hero or heroine as tomorrow's flop; today's crush on a new girlfriend or boyfriend may fade overnight.

Parents can assist the adolescent in achieving self-regulation and self-mastery. Although the adolescent "separates" in that he or she seems to rely less and less on parental ministrations, adolescent-parent ties have simply changed. Parents are still important parts of silently operating psychological structures. Studies of competently functioning adolescents and youth consistently validate the importance of psychological ties to parents (Stein et al. 1987). The adolescent reworks these ties and transforms them psychologically. He or she loosens primitive attachments through to-and-fro attachment-detachment behavior with peers and newly found love relationships. The adolescent gradually develops an internal competence to function without the physical presence of the parents, without conscious awareness of their importance. The adolescent achieves cohesion, an experience of inner homeostasis, as he or she modifies the nature of ties to parents, increasingly turns to peers and others for the kind of sustenance needed, and in later adolescence and young adulthood, develops psychological skills for which he or she will be noted for the rest of life. Fragmentation of this process threatens self-sustenance or the bonds that sustain oneself. The adolescent may experience a sense of "falling apart," a sense of inner emptiness, or some sort of painful disruption of smooth functioning. Such fragmentation may often appear in a suicidal wish, plan, or attempt.

Adolescence is a time of special vulnerability to injuries to self-esteem and disappointments in valued persons. How well teenagers have been able to sustain themselves with old and new personal relationships and with their own psychological functioning determines how painful or how disruptive these injuries and disappointments, real or imagined, will be. Shame or rage may result when the adolescents no longer feel powerful or when their attachment to an idealized other is thwarted. Shame and rage are complex emotions, which often include intolerable somatic responses that may lead to suicidal behavior. Shame and rage may result from how adolescents perceive their experiences with others, not always from how others actually behave. Nonetheless, the behavior of others does have its impact.

Relational Aspects of Development

The normal adolescent separation and distancing from parents in no way negates continuing parental influences, even though adolescents may deny them or be unaware of their strength. Part of the real world milieu for adolescents is their parents' valuation and respect for their evolving autonomy and individual identity. How well do parents tolerate the adolescent's healthy need to question and struggle against them? Are the parents confident enough to offer guidance and to set limits when adolescent rebellion or exploration threatens to become genuinely self-damaging, and are they knowledgeable and sensitive enough to recognize that distinction?

Parents are the most powerful objects of identification and role models at the core of a youngster's identity. Much of an adolescent's capacity to cope with stress will have been built from observing and internalizing the parents' responses and their use of resources during difficult times. Parents' relationships with each other and with extended family and friends shape a child's expectations of support from peers and from the wider community. Parents' integration into their own microculture and into the dominant culture is crucially determinative of the young person's internal optimism or pessimism about his or her capacity to belong and to find a psychologically comfortable place in the world. Parental psycho-pathology is deeply distortive of the emotional resources that a child brings to the tasks and stresses of adolescence.

The family systems perspective on health and dysfunction views the family as an interactional whole composed of sets of patterned rela-tionships and communication processes that reflect the particular family's unique organization and structure. These relationships and pro-cesses produce ways of functioning that may either facilitate or inhibit the developmental trajectories across the life cycle of the family and its individual members (McGoldrick and Walsh 1983). Causality is viewed as circular, complex, and the product of multiple influences and inter-dependent processes. Thus, the influence of life events is mediated by multiple variables—meanings, relationships, contexts—most impor-tantly the family's organizational patterns and coping responses (Bateson 1972; Hoffman 1981). Symptoms in the individual family member are seen as an expression of family dysfunction, an inability to respond adaptively to external stress and developmental challenge while pro-viding protection and nurturance to family members.

Stress is inherent in all development and change, and most particu-larly during periods of family transition across the life cycle. One such transition is adolescence. Transitional periods pose adaptive challenges for the family system (Walsh and Scheinkman 1993). Each new transi-tion involves structural reorganization and the renegotiation of relation-ship rules and roles (Hoffman 1988). These periods are characterized by disequilibrium in the family system, where family stability and conti-nuity are perturbed by the pressures for change. It is at these periods of destabilization that families and individual members are likely to be-come symptomatic. When life cycle transitions reawaken unresolved issues from earlier transitional stresses, they are likely to be more com-plex and to contribute to dysfunction. This is particularly true of the adolescent stage, when family functioning must change to provide a context in which the adolescent may accomplish the developmental tasks of that stage.

Adaptations in family organization are essential to meet the devel-opmental tasks of adolescence. These adaptive processes transform the family from a unit geared to protect, nurture, and socialize the young child, into one that prepares the adolescent for an adult world of re-sponsibilities and commitments (Garcia-Preto 1988). Three major tasks of adolescence—sexuality with the transformation of the physical self, identity formation, and autonomy—produce a disequilibrium and a normal challenge that the family must master by accommodative change. Conversely, the stability of family structure provides a "holding environment" within which the adolescent may reorganize around biological, cognitive, and social changes.

Sexuality and the transformation of the physical self precipitated by the biological processes of puberty require a renegotiation within the family of issues of physical contact, expressions of affection, boundaries, and privacy. Emerging adolescent sexuality demands a new level of openness and directness as parents and adolescents discuss the adolescent's sexuality and related topics in an atmosphere of acceptance. This new sexuality has a profound effect on boundary issues within the family, leading to a developmentally appropriate clarification of generational boundaries and role distinctions. Thus, the manner in which the family responds to adolescent sexuality—its beliefs, attitudes, affects, and behaviors—can either foster or impair the mastery and integration of impulse and feeling and either positively or negatively influence the emotional coloring of this central aspect of an adolescent's life.

Identity formation involves those psychological processes of differentiation of the self from the family matrix, exploration of new relationships, and the development of a more complex perception of the self, others, and the social world. These complex processes seem to occur in a developmental dialectic in which adolescent identity is begun in opposition to parental values and beliefs, opposition being the ground from which difference may be constructed. From behavioral opposition, through cognitive differences of belief and value, to a differentiation that represents a synthesis of similarities (identifications) and differences, the adolescent and family traverse a long and difficult path toward a reunion as adults within a new set of relationships. Required of the family during this adventure is stability, flexibility, and support. Hauser et al. (1984) have reported research that has shown that family interactions emphasizing warmth, acceptance, and understanding tend to support higher levels of ego development and identity formation in the adolescent family member.

The development of autonomy by the adolescent requires balancing by the family of ongoing limit-setting functions and appropriate opportunities for independent activity and exploration. This balance will lead to the development of judgment, decision-making skills, and an interest in the novel and the new. Families that provide too little (permissive) or too much (rigid) supervision, structure, or containment seem to contribute to increased risk of adolescent acting out of conflicts. Optimum containment maintains connectedness, and optimum connectedness provides a secure space for exploration and autonomy. Adolescence threatens previous attachments, precipitates feelings of loss and fears of abandonment, and requires renegotiation and rebalancing of attachment relationships.

The effective functioning of the family in response to the stress of the adolescent transition may be conceptualized along several key dimensions (Walsh and Scheinkman 1993):

- Adaptability is seen as the family's ability to balance between maintaining a stable structure and allowing for flexibility in response to developmental challenge. This is particularly true of the family's need to respond flexibly to the adolescent's developmental need for increasing autonomy and responsibility while continuing to provide consistent and stable structures. Dysfunction in this dimension is characterized by rigidity or chaos with resulting acting-out and risk-taking.
- Cohesion is seen as the family's ability to balance needs for closeness and connectedness versus respect for separateness, privacy, and difference. In adolescence it becomes necessary for the family to move from what Sterlin (1974) has called a centripetal pattern, a pull inward, to a centrifugal pattern of interaction and structure that pushes out, supporting the differentiation of adolescent family members. Dysfunction in this dimension may lead to enmeshment, where families hold on and make it difficult for individuation to develop, where families hurry emotional distancing and separation producing pseudoindependence and incomplete ego development. Well-functioning families are respectful of individual boundaries between parents and children associated with age-appropriate privileges and responsibilities and maintain a clear sense of family–community boundary that defines the family as a unit open to the larger social community.
- Affect regulation and communication is seen as the family's capacity to balance a need to regulate, modulate, and contain affects with support for the articulation and expression of each family member's subjective experiences. This balance requires the family's respect for varying levels of competence at affective expression, particularly during the adolescent transition, as well as tolerance of increased aggression and lability. Dysfunction in this dimension is

characterized by family patterns of externalization, such as critical, blaming, scapegoating interactions, and an absence of the empathy, interest, and warmth necessary for mutual problem solving and trust.

Peer relations and influences can be (although often only for the short term) more powerful than that of parents. The turn to the peer group is not only a defensive withdrawal from parents, it is a healthy move into a social milieu that will continue into the future to constitute the bulk of one's interpersonal world. A basic issue at times of crisis is the sense of being an insider or an outsider; does the adolescent fit in with some sufficiently valued peer group and thus have access to some psychological support?

One's peer group status usually varies over time for each adolescent. Identity is evolving and changing, and most adolescents try on for size a number of differing identities. An adolescent's drift toward a specific peer group, or the shift to successive peer groups, reveals something of what is going on intrapsychically in that particular youngster. Thus, the psychological importance of the peer group is also a function of the adolescent's choice, not only the group's influence on the teenager. In this process, peer group aspirations and identifications shift, so that not only may there be different degrees of success or failure in the sense of peer group acceptance and support, but each shift also entails the loss of social supports and perhaps a period of temporary isolation.

Some shifts of peer group are not entirely of the adolescent's choosing. The youngster who leaves home for the military or prep school or college usually does so voluntarily—even eagerly—but he or she is not knowingly choosing the individuals in that new peer group. There are separation concerns regardless of how fervently the youngster yearns for this new freedom. It is often a shock to discover that one has gone from being a big fish in the somewhat limited and familiar peer group(s) at home, to being a little fish in a vast new environment. In addition, the freedom itself is a mixed blessing. Sexual freedom and the free opportunity to indulge in abusable substances away from immediate parental awareness are stresses for which many newly fledged students and recruits are both unprepared and incapable of withstanding.

Each peer group has its own characteristics in terms of its preferred coping techniques and shared adaptive or maladaptive mechanisms, its values, its future orientation, its integration into or isolation from the imminent adult world, and its capacity to provide nurturance and support to its members when needed. These qualities in one's group influence the outcome when an individual youngster faces a perceived crisis that seems to render the value of living questionable.

In the special area of sexual identity development, the crucial element of the sense of self and self-worth is highly dependent on its valuation and validation by others. Parents' responses to their child's sexual maturation set the stage for sociosexual entry into the peer group. Even before active sexuality begins, one's peers, the social response to one's maleness or femaleness, and one's unique masculinity or femininity, has an immense impact on self-confidence. Particularly at this formative stage, one's partner of choice plays a major role in the adolescent's sexual validation. Adolescents often despair if their finding someone to love and to be loved by lags behind the experience of their peers.

There is a built-in and virtually inevitable source of loss, as well as gain, in this aspect of adolescent development. Keeping, marrying, and living happily with one's first love is a rare experience. The instability of adolescent identity means repetitive change and loss of love partners. Yet each love is real and intense, and each loss is potentially devastating. It is not suggested that remaining with one's first love is the ideal course for development. Most first loves occur when the adolescents are grossly immature; they have yet no idea of what their own adult identities will be or what kind of personality in a partner will best fit them. However, loss is a factor in suicide risk at all ages, and especially for those who by definition lack a maturely developed inner sense of self-worth and security and who still find it difficult to see beyond the realities and emotions of the moment. Problems with and losses of girlfriends and boyfriends are a frequent precursor of adolescent suicide.

Adolescents with atypical gender identities or sexual orientation are in an especially vulnerable position. Although tolerance for variations from species-typical heterosexual orientation varies from peer group to peer group, as well as from culture to culture, nowhere are obvious variations accorded equal status, especially among adolescents, and it is during adolescence that deviations from the norms most often become conscious to the individual and apparent to others. *Confusion* and *self-loathing* are frequent, if not typical, and are compounded by isolation when there is peer rejection. *Suicide* and *suicidal ideation* are high among adolescents (especially males) upon newly discovering a homosexual orientation. The full impact of transsexualism comes predictably in adolescence, and attempted and completed suicide rates are very high among transsexuals (Gibson 1989; Harry 1989).

Sociocultural Factors
in Adolescent Development

Some of the phenomenological aspects of cultural influences were discussed in Chapter 1. The relevance in terms of development is twofold: 1) How do specific cultural institutions, childrearing philosophies, and expectations integrate with what adolescents need for normal or optimal development? and 2) Within any given culture, what accounts for the fact that although some adolescents attempt or complete suicide, most do not?

With regard to the first question, examples from Chapter 1 can be informative. The Japanese seem to compromise individuality and isolate adolescents from any sense of a supportive network of peers. Danish culture, too, ties adolescents to maternal expectations, while emotional expressiveness and release or angry rebelliousness is discouraged. For Danish youngsters, paternal support is also poor, and the highly urban culture makes for a milieu of social strangers. The intense competitiveness in Sweden, also true in Japan and Denmark, has the effect of forcing preferred aspects of identity onto adolescents and undervaluing those for whom these requirements do not fit. By contrast, Norway's lesser focus on competition allows for greater acceptance of individual differences. Both its childrearing philosophies and its ecology provide and encourage family and social supports during personal and social difficulties.

Most industrialized cultures foster thinking about the consequences of actions through their educational institutions. However, in any large culture such as the Judeo-Christian, its achievement varies enormously according to actual quality of education, subcultural and ethnic differences in emphasis, and status and familial differences in what is valued. A striking example is seen in the threefold higher teenage pregnancy rate in the United States when compared with all other developed countries. Studies by the Guttmacher Institute (E. F. Jones et al. 1985) found that the most significant determinant of the difference was the pervading philosophy regarding adolescent intercourse. In the countries with the lower rate, the focus is on avoiding the damaging consequences of intercourse, principally pregnancy. In the United States, the focus is on the prevention of intercourse. In the one case, the overall cultural philosophy both recognizes the reality of adolescent sexuality and actively fosters thinking about consequences; in the other the culture denies and tries to change reality, while deemphasizing the imperativeness of thinking of consequences.

Disrupted cultures and disadvantaged subcultural groups are more likely to fail adolescents in all areas of providing for healthy needs and for opportunities to fulfill adolescent tasks. Families are more often dysfunctional and convey a sense of hopelessness. Such circumstances provide a poorer preparation for adolescence, as well as a less advantageous family and cultural milieu during adolescence. If the subculture was originally a simple nonindustrial one, there is less traditional background for fostering propositional thought in ways necessary for successful function in a technological culture, although the potential for such development exists in the normal brain. The realities facing adolescents in these conditions are genuinely bleaker, thus requiring even stronger, rather than compromised, adolescents to cope effectively. Disadvantaged circumstances lead to a high incidence of sociocultural (self-destruction in terms of function within one's culture) as well as actual suicide.

With regard to suicidal variability within cultures, some cultural designations can be so broad (Western culture, Judeo-Christian culture) as to preclude all but the most general uniformities. Smaller subcultural groups within even more limited cultural entities may, for example, have markedly different childrearing patterns than those of the larger culture. From a clinical standpoint, suicidal variations within even small, reasonably homogeneous cultures are as compelling of interest as are cross-cultural differences.

Although cultural institutions, including childrearing practices and typical patterns of family interactions, grow out of shared psychodynamics, these institutions do not affect all groups and families identically. Some cultural expectations are not accepted by some individual families. Some parents openly reject majority opinions regarding childrearing and relationships with adolescents. They may have been exposed to and be aware of alternative ways of preparing children for adolescence and adulthood.

In a pathogenic or disrupted culture some families may be unusually healthy and functional. For reasons that may not yet be understood they may be able to rise above dismal realities and provide their adolescents with a durable inner sense of worth and loveability. One may speculate that this is the major basis of an effective and healthy adolescence under generally adverse circumstances.

There are many dysfunctional families and unconstructive peer groups even in potentially health-promoting cultures. The destructive influences, especially in early parent-child interactions, can be very subtle, as shown by Stern's (1985) research involving frequent, repetitive "micro-moments" of parental influence. Finally, there are individual genetic and constitutional differences between adolescents that are not culturally determined (see Chapter 3).

In summary, although the framework of different cultures puts adolescents at generally differential suicide risk, the occurrence of actual or sociocultural suicide within that culture probably depends on

- The influence of the individual's family of rearing on the preparation of the adolescent for the tasks of adolescence and for the adolescent and adult realities to be faced and on the essential core self-perception as being loveable and valuable,
- The values and qualities of the adolescent's particular peer group at the time of crisis, and
- The possibility of some biological factors that have a role in individual resistance or vulnerability to either eugenic or pathogenic family or cultural influences.

3

Research Into Suicidality

Epidemiology

Epidemiology concerns itself with the rates and the distribution of a condition in the population as well as with the factors associated with it. Here we are concerned with suicidal behaviors and completed suicide in adolescence. Adolescent suicide refers to such events occurring between puberty and adulthood. The National Center for Health Statistics and the World Health Organization use an age grouping of 15–19 years, but this excludes the important group of early adolescents.

Rates and Distribution

Many methodological problems exist in the epidemiological study of adolescent suicide, the most salient of which is underreporting. The suicide of a young person has an overwhelming impact on family, friends, and the community. It may be covered up intentionally because of guilt, religious reasons, or social stigma. Other violent deaths (e.g., death by homicide or accidental death) may involve a suicidal intent that is impossible to ascertain. Homicide and accidents can be more subtle manifestations of self-destructive tendencies and risk-taking (Holinger and Klemen 1982).

Ellen, a 16-year-old girl, was seen as an emergency after she had stolen
her parent's car and driven it into a telephone pole. She had been in therapy
previously for depression and immediately prior to the accident she had
argued with her parents about their wish that she return to therapy. Her
previous depression had improved with therapy, but they were concerned
about a return of poor self-esteem, deteriorating academic performance,
social isolation, irritability, and sleep disturbance. She had escaped the
accident with only minor injuries. She admitted the return of depressive
symptomatology to the psychiatrist but denied suicidal ideation or intent
behind the accident.[1]

Had the accident in the above vignette been fatal one cannot be sure
how it should be classified. A further problem is that the relative rarity
of this event makes the evaluation of risk factors, and specifically the
evaluation of causality, an almost impossible endeavor.

It is fortunate that completed adolescent suicide is indeed a rare
event. Although considerably more common than prepubertal suicide,
adolescent suicide is about 10 times less common than during subsequent stages of life. In the younger age groups, rates increase dramatically after puberty and peak at age 23 (Shaffer and Fisher 1981). The rate
for the population as a whole gradually increases after that age. The
marked increase during the adult years is specifically attributable to a
marked increase occurring in elderly men. The rates of suicide among
15- to 19-year-olds in the United States have increased over the past
four decades; a steady increase was observed from 1960 (3.6 deaths/
100,000) through 1970 (5.9/100,000) and 1980 (8.5/100,000) to 1990 (11.1/
100,000) (National Center for Health Statistics 1963, 1974, 1985, 1994).
Suicide ranks second only to accidents as the leading cause of death in
late adolescence (Rosenberg et al. 1987). Holinger and Offer (1982) noted
that during the 20th century, although changes in the total number of
adolescent suicides increased or decreased with fluctuations in the numbers and proportions of adolescents in the population, the *rates* of
adolescent suicide (deaths/100,000 population) have increased indepen-
dently of the total numbers. An absolute increase has occurred in the

---

[1]In this report, all identifying indications of ethnic or racial background and
socioeconomic status have been purposefully omitted from all vignettes, except
for what may be inevitably inferred from the essential facts of a vignette. The
cases cited throughout the report are drawn from many different backgrounds
and from various clinical settings, ranging from inner-city emergency departments to private practice. A previous Group for the Advancement of Psychiatry
report (1989) focused specifically on the relevance of culture and ethnicity to
suicide.

adolescent population in the past decades and thus an increase in both the total number and in the rates of adolescent suicide. The latter finding represents a true increase because mortality rates as defined are not expected to increase with an increase in population (Holinger and Offer 1989). Others have demonstrated a cohort effect in the increase in suicide rates among the young (Murphy and Wetzel 1980; Solomon and Hellon 1980). The findings of these investigators indicate that both in the United States and Canada each successive birth cohort started with a higher suicide rate and that at successive 5-year intervals each birth cohort had a higher rate than the preceding cohort had at the same age. Both models of analysis indicate that the increase in both the rate and the absolute number of adolescent suicide over the past decades is real.

There is evidence to suggest that not only has the rate of completed suicides increased, but that the frequency of *attempted* suicide has also dramatically increased over the past two decades (Harkavy-Friedman et al. 1987; K. Smith and Crawford 1986). The prevalence of suicidal behavior among high school students is approximately 9%, and an estimated 2 million 15- to 24-year-olds attempt suicide every year. Evidently, suicidal gestures or attempts are serious behaviors that cannot be disregarded or trivialized simply because of their frequent occurrence. Higher rates have been noted for completed suicides among previous attempters, and increased rates of previous attempts have been found among completed suicides (Gould et al. 1990, 1992). Parasuicidal behavior is considered to be a decided risk factor for completed suicide. In this report, parasuicide refers to behavior, not ideation or intent; any action from a subtle gesture to a true suicide attempt that failed is considered parasuicide (Coombs et al. 1992).

A continuing controversy in the field of suicidology has been how to characterize and label suicidal behavior. The generic term *suicidal behavior* includes completed suicide, parasuicidal behavior (e.g., suicide attempts or suicide gestures), suicide communications including suicide threats, and suicidal ideation. Suicidal ideation is so common that it may be considered a normal phenomenon (Pfeffer et al. 1984). Whitaker and Shaffer (1993) found that 40% of a total population of 5,000 teenagers from a rural area entertained suicidal ideas, whereas only 5% had ever made a suicide attempt. Bolger et al. (1989) in a retrospective questionnaire study of 364 college students found that suicidal thoughts in childhood are typical and that the risk of such thoughts begins to increase by age 9 years.

Researchers do not agree whether those who complete suicide and those who make nonfatal suicide attempts constitute a single or perhaps several distinct populations. Shaffer et al. (1988) observed that parasuicide is usually a nonlethal behavior, shown predominantly by young females who take a nonlethal overdose of a potentially poisonous substance but who do not wish to die. After an extensive literature review, Linehan (1986) concluded that parasuicides are a heterogeneous group. Group differences, she believed, are congruent with the hypothesis that the serious parasuicides where the wish to die and medical risk are high consists of persons who belong in either the suicide population or one that overlaps it substantially. In this report, we differentiate suicidal ideation from suicidal attempts (whether manipulative, a cry for help, or a series of uncompleted attempts) and from completed suicide, and we address essentially physical self-damage rather than the many other ways adolescents can place themselves at serious disadvantage.

The preferred method for completed adolescent suicide for both boys and girls in the United States is firearms (Boyd and Moscicki 1986). The next most common method for boys is hanging, whereas for girls it is jumping from a height (Shaffer et al. 1988). Brent et al. (1987) noted evidence of higher rates of substance abuse among suicide victims who used firearms as their method. An overdose of drugs or other medications—the most common method of suicide among adults—is seldom used by teenagers.

Sexual, ethnic, and geographic differences exist in rates of completed adolescent suicides in the United States; close to five times more teenage boys complete suicide than do girls, and the rates in whites are higher than in nonwhites although not necessarily higher than in Amerind adolescents. Shaffer et al. (1988) have noted that the sex differences appear to be considerably less marked among Hispanics and somewhat less so among blacks. In contrast to completed adolescent suicides, unsuccessful suicides are four times more common in females than in males. Geography also seems to have some relationship to the rate of adolescent suicide in the United States. The rates are highest in western states and Alaska and lower in the eastern states (Vital Statistics of the U.S. 1984).

Risk Factors

Carl, a 15-year-old boy, was brought to the emergency room by his maternal grandmother who was worried about his talk that everything would be better if he were dead and who may have seen him looking for his mother's gun. Carl had not seen his father since his parents' divorce 10 years earlier and lived with his grandmother and mother. His mother had a history of psychotic depression and was emotionally unavailable to him. Carl had no friends and recounted that others disliked and avoided him. He knew of a recent suicide attempt by a school peer and he described a clear plan for how he would kill himself with the gun. Despite no history of prior suicide attempts, Carl was hospitalized because of the presence of several severe suicide risk factors: family history of depression, little family support, high lethality of chosen suicide method, knowledge of suicide attempt by a peer, and peer rejection.

Sudak et al. (1984) attribute the steady increase of youth suicide in recent decades to increasing social disintegration evidenced by increased divorce rates or the diminishing importance of religious and moral values. The loosening of social cohesion presumably contributes to personal alienation and thereby to increased suicide potential. Among students, those who commit suicide gave evidence of not being well integrated into their social groups and college students seemed more likely to commit suicide than their non-student-age peers (Huffine 1989).

More specific and immediate social stresses have an impact on adolescent suicidality. The data of Shaffer et al. (1988) on completed suicides suggest that many teenagers commit suicide in the context of an acute disciplinary crisis or shortly after a rejection or humiliation and that there is but a brief interval between the acute stress and the suicide attempt. In their study on adolescent suicide attempters, Tischler et al. (1981) similarly found that the most frequently cited precipitants were family problems, problems with the opposite sex, and school problems. In that study only half of the sample were living at home with both parents at the time of the event.

Although social stresses have been associated with both completed and attempted suicides, these cannot be considered as sufficient causes by themselves. The rates and frequency of stressful circumstances (e.g., family breakdown or loss) are similar in the lives of both nondisturbed and disturbed adolescents who do not attempt suicide suggesting that the phenomena are not specific to the suicidal adolescent (Paykel 1989). Stressful circumstances and events seem to interact with other personality variables as well as with personal and familial psychopathology to lead to suicidality.

In a comparison of adolescent suicide attempters with both depressed and nondepressed adolescents who had never attempted suicide, de Wilde et al. (1992) found that ". . . the suicide attempt seems embedded not just in the problems every adolescent has to deal with but in greater turmoil in their families, rooted in childhood and not stabilizing in adolescence, in combination with traumatic events during adolescence and social instability in the year preceding the attempt" (p. 45).

Shafii (1989) distinguished completed adolescent suicides from attempts along a number of parameters. In contrast to attempters, completers had been exposed to the suicide of a parent, adult relative, sibling, or friend; their parents had significant emotional problems and had either been absent or abusive; they had expressed suicidal ideation or made a suicidal threat or a previous suicide attempt; they frequently used drugs and alcohol, engaged in antisocial behavior, and demonstrated an inhibited personality; and they had received previous psychiatric treatment. Shafii concluded that suicide is not an impulsive act, but a response to a "final straw" in a long history of serious and chronic emotional and behavioral problems.

Shaffer et al. (1988) reported that approximately half of their completed suicides had had previous contact with a mental health professional for a variety of problems, including depression, antisocial behavior, drug and alcohol abuse, and learning disorders. A high proportion of the suicide completers had a first- or second-degree relative who had previously attempted or completed suicide. Even higher rates of other psychopathology (92%) are reported in the "under 30" completed suicide group in the San Diego suicide study (C. L. Rich et al. 1986).

Nevertheless, conflicting reports exist in the literature. Carlson and Cantwell (1982), in a study of referred children and adolescents, reported that attempters do not differ from nonattempters in any particular diagnostic category. Sexual identity issues and sexual problems are associated with higher rates of suicidality; these include homosexuality, confusion over sexual identity, sexual victimization, and teenage pregnancy (Gibson 1989; Harry 1989). Although the more common disorders associated with increased suicidality are affective disorders, substance abuse during the course of these disorders can increase the vulnerability to suicide.

C. L. Rich et al. (1988) examined the relationship between the most common psychiatric illnesses and the most common stressors in 283 suicides. They found that interpersonal loss or conflicts, medical illness, and economic problems were most common and occurred more frequently near the time of death for substance abusers with and without depression than for persons with "pure" affective disorders. Murphy et al. (1979) found that frequent interpersonal loss (26%) clustered 6 weeks prior to death. Rosen (1976) described the most common risk factors as living alone, unemployment, psychosis, alcohol or drug abuse, sudden life changes, loss of a parent, family history of suicide, and past suicide attempts. Blumenthal and Kupfer (1986) reported similar findings.

The risk factors most prominently noted by Pallis et al. (1982) were being male, younger than 45, from a low socioeconomic status, depressed, unemployed, living alone, abusing alcohol, and speaking of suicide. Brent et al. (1988) considered the most significant stressor to be substance abuse. Other contributing factors noted by Brent et al. were a suicide act with high intent, violent method, exposure to suicidal behavior, a family history of affective disorder, and access to firearms. Gould et al. (1990) found risk factors that are particularly important as predictors of adolescent suicide are prior suicide attempt (increasing the risk over 20 times that for a comparison group of males), diagnosis of depression, use of drugs and alcohol, antisocial behavior, and having a family member who exhibited suicidal behavior.

Access to firearms is a frequently mentioned risk factor and has been the object of intense controversy. The evidence supporting the availability of firearms as a risk factor for suicide has been derived largely from ecological studies (i.e., studies based on aggregate data for entire communities, states, or even countries correlating various indicators of firearm availability with suicide rates). Some of these studies have found a correlation between various measures of gun availability and both firearm and total suicide rates (Boor and Bair 1990; Boyd and Moscicki 1986; Cantor and Lewin 1990; Killias 1993; Lester 1989). Others suggest a relationship with firearm suicide rates but not with total suicide rates suggesting that when firearms are not available, other methods are substituted (Clarke and Jones 1989; Lester 1990; Sloan et al. 1990). Studies examining the impact of gun control laws on suicide rates also have had conflicting results (Lester and Murrel 1982; Loftin et al. 1991; C. L. Rich et al. 1990; Sloan et al. 1990). One of these studies found that although restricting access to handguns did not reduce the overall suicide rate, it was associated with a reduced overall rate among adolescents and young adults ages 15–24 years, suggesting that method substitution may be less likely to occur in adolescents and young adults (Sloan et al. 1990).

A significant limitation of ecological studies such as those cited above, is the aggregate nature of the data and therefore the difficulty in assessing the role that availability of guns might have in each individual suicide. Case control studies have been used more recently in an effort to address this problem. Several such studies of adolescent suicide victims have found the availability of handguns in the home to be a significant risk factor for suicide in this age group (Brent et al. 1988, 1991, 1993; Kellerman et al. 1992). Kellerman et al. (1992) studied all suicides in two United States counties that took place at home and matched each suicide victim with a control subject from the same neighborhood of the same sex, race, and age range. The relationship between ready availability of firearms in the home and an increased risk of suicide held even after statistically controlling for several potentially confounding variables (e.g., drug and alcohol use; history of depression or mental illness). These data have been cited to suggest that guns somehow stimulate a suicidal wish and "cause" suicide, but evidence for such causality and the nature of a corresponding dynamic motivation is not available. Although, as indicated by research cited above, much of adolescent suicide is not a sudden impulse, there are some indications that impulsivity and substance abuse may play a more prominent role in youthful suicide than in older groups (Brent et al. 1987; Dudley et al. 1992; C. L. Rich et al. 1986; Shaffer 1993). If this is so, it could be an explanation for the finding that availability of a gun may play a more critical role in determining suicide rates among youth than in older adults.

Biological Factors

The likelihood of suicide depends on the interplay of innate as well as environmental factors. *Innate* factors include both genetic predisposition as well as specific biochemical abnormalities (serotonin, dopamine, or norepiphrine metabolism). *Environmental* factors include intrauterine, perinatal, and family stressors and a history of psychic trauma. It is important that the clinician distinguish between depressed adolescents who are dysthymic because of a reaction to psychosocial stressors (i.e., death of a parent or showing the effects of living with a depressed parent) and ones who are demonstrating specific vulnerability to affective disorder.

Genetic Factors

The following case clearly involves both environmental and genetic factors; it is used here because of the genetic component.

> Michael, a 15-year-old male, was brought to the emergency room by his mother and stepfather. They had been notified by the school counselor

that he had shown friends a gun he had brought to school with which to kill himself. The counselor was further concerned because there had been a recent suicide by another student. There was a history of severe alcohol abuse by both his mother and stepfather, and his biological father had a history of severe mood swings and had been hospitalized several times for serious suicide attempts. Michael had been deeply embarrassed and compromised the previous evening when his mother had overheard him talking to a friend about selling some marijuana and had turned the names of his friends over to the police. He expressed a serious wish to die and had a plan for suicide. His mother was totally unsupportive and bitter, complaining that Michael was just like his father, only wanted attention, and saying that if he really wanted to kill himself he would have done so by now.

In past years genetic hypotheses for suicide were infrequent. The Kallmann and Anastasio (1947) twin studies for example found high concordance rates for major psychiatric disorders but no concordance for suicide and concluded that genetic factors did not play a significant role. Subsequently, Juel-Nielsen and Videbach (1970) found that a significant number of monozygotic twins had committed suicide. A highly significant concentration was noted of suicide occurring in biological relatives of adoptees who had either committed suicide or who had a major depressive disorder (the adoptees had not been exposed to their biological family environment). In a Danish study of adopted twins living apart, Schulsinger et al. (1979) found a 4.5% incidence of suicide in biological relatives of adoptees who had committed suicide compared with 1% in the biological relatives of the comparison group. (There were no suicides in the adoptive relatives of either group.)

There is evidence that severe depression plus multiple suicides in some family lines and severe depression without suicide in other family lines may reflect separable genetic populations. There may be different genetic factors in repetitive familial suicidality than in depression alone (Roy 1991).

Tsuang (1983) and Roy (1983) both found significantly higher rates for suicidal behavior in the families of patients who committed suicide than in control groups. Thus a genetic predisposition to suicide may exist although evidence from genetic studies is inconclusive—perhaps the genetic predisposition for impulse-dyscontrol and depression in an individual challenged by stressful life circumstances can result in suicidal behavior.

There is consistent evidence supporting the role, however, of a genetically transmitted vulnerability to affective and especially bipolar disorder (Tsuang 1978). Major depression is a heritable, recurrent syndromal illness (Gold et al. 1988). The authors observed that before drug treatment became available, studies of depressed patients consistently showed suicide rates of 30% and at least a 30% incidence of serious attempts. A high proportion of suicide completers had a first- or second-degree relative who had previously attempted or committed suicide (Shaffer and Gould 1987).

The cyclic nature of bipolar disorder and the genetic predisposition were noted by Kraepelin (1913). Gershon et al. (1987) determined that for the child of one bipolar parent the risk of bipolar disorder is 27%, whereas the risk figure for the child with two bipolar parents is from 50% to 75%. Twin studies also suggest a genetic contribution for major depression and bipolar disorder. Bertelson et al. (1975) found that 65% of monozygotic twins in their sample were concordant for major affective disorder compared with 14% of dizygotic twins. Although definite genetic markers have not yet been found, genetic linkage studies point to several chromosomal abnormalities (chromosome 11 and an X-linked chromosome) in bipolar patients.

Neuroendocrine Factors

Unlike studies of suicidal behavior, many studies have explored the biological basis of major depressive disorder. To elucidate the biological underpinnings of affective disorders in childhood, research strategies similar to those used with adults have been applied.

Abnormalities of cortisol secretion are found in a significant subgroup of adults with endogenous depressions in whom this finding represents a marker of the acute depressive episode—a marker of state rather than trait. Studies of endogenously depressed prepubertal children have found that approximately 20%, a rate about half that found in adults, are cortisol hypersecretors (Puig-Antich et al. 1983). The dexamethasone suppression test (DST) has been used to identify a group of adult depressive patients who fail to show normal pituitary suppression after its administration. Similar findings have been reported in endogenously depressed prepubertal children. However, the diagnostic value of the DST in children and adolescents is limited because of an apparent lack of specificity (Shaffer 1985).

Abnormal secretion of growth hormone has been found in some endogenously depressed children (Puig-Antich et al. 1983). Both hyposecretion in response to the insulin tolerance test and hypersecretion during sleep were presumed to result from a disturbance of hypothalamic serotonin mechanisms. These abnormalities also were found to be present after recovery from the acute depressed episodes which suggests that they could represent a trait as well as a state marker.

Putative abnormalities of central biogenic amine systems figure prominently in current biological models of the pathophysiology of affective disorders. Similar to findings in adults, chronically depressed children have been found to excrete lower levels of MHPG (3-methoxy, 4 hydroxy phenylglycol) in their urine than do control subjects (Cytryn et al. 1984). The tendency for some depressed adults and adolescents to reverse polarity and exhibit a hypomanic response to the administration of amines and tricyclics is consistent with the biogenic amine hypothesis of affective disorders. That this response may represent a trait marker for bipolar illness was found to be 100% specific in identifying those depressed adolescents who would later go on to show a bipolar course (Akiskal et al. 1985). Similar responses to tricyclics and stimulants are well known in childhood, but no follow-up studies of these children have been reported.

Dysfunction of the central serotonergic system (5-HT) has been associated with major depression (Meltzer and Lowy 1987). The likelihood that the serotonin system is also associated with suicidal or impulsive aggressive behavior has been postulated by Asberg et al. (1976) who found low concentrations of the serotonin metabolite 5-hydroxyindoleacetic acid (5-HIAA) in the cerebrospinal fluid (CSF) of suicide attempters and completers. G. L. Brown et al. (1982) and Stanley and Mann (1988) found alterations in serotonin metabolism in aggressive men with borderline personality disorder. The CNS 5-HIAA levels were significantly lower in the subjects who had a history of suicide than in those who have not been suicidal. 5-HIAA has been found to be lower in concentration in the CSF of patients who attempted suicide in a violent manner (firearms) than in those who attempted suicide in a less violent manner (drugs). A low concentration of 5-HIAA in CSF has been found in patients with disorders of impulsivity, including arsonists, violent offenders, and alcoholic patients (Asberg et al. 1987; Ballenger et al. 1979; G. L. Brown et al. 1982; Kaplan and Sadock 1991; Roy 1989; Virkkunen et al. 1987). McElroy et al. (1992) studied group impulse control disorders with other forms of affective spectrum disorders, all of which may share an abnormality in serotonin transmission. A low concentration of 5-HIAA in CSF has been found in children and adolescents who have a history of aggression and impulsive behavior (Kruesi 1989; Kruesi et al. 1990).

Coccaro et al. (1989) noted the difficulty in attributing these findings to impulsive aggression alone because low 5-HIAA was found to be decreased in individuals with a variety of diagnoses, including persons with *major* depressive disorders, those with borderline personality disorders, suicide attemptors, and criminal offenders, as well as nonpsychiatric volunteers. Their study suggested that self-directed and other-directed aggressive–impulsive behaviors are associated with reduced 5-HT function not accounted for by confounding factors such as a history of major affective disorder or alcohol abuse. In other words, they believe there is a psychobiological basis for aggressive-impulsive behavior and that reduced 5-HT metabolism is related to aggression (auto) rather than depression. Van Praag et al. (1986), however, hypothesized that both mood and aggressive disorders are related to lowered 5-HT. This hypothesis, they believe, is consistent with the clinical observation that disorders in mood and aggression go hand in hand.

Psychiatric and Psychological Factors

Relation to psychiatric disorders.

Joel, a 17-year-old male, had been referred to outpatient individual and group psychotherapy for what appeared to be minor suicide gestures and for difficulties in relating to his divorced parents and his stepparents. He also had many fantasies of shooting himself and unspecified others "to get back at them." There were several crisis hospitalizations during therapy until his completed suicide. He had been seen by his therapist the evening before his suicide and had said, "See you in group tomorrow" on leaving. The next morning he shot himself in the head in front of one of his classes at school. It was reported that he had made a suicide pact with a friend (who did not commit suicide), of which he had not informed his therapist. His diagnosis had been major depression and personality disorder not otherwise specified, with many borderline, antisocial, and passive-aggressive features.

There is general agreement among researchers that there is a high prevalence of psychiatric disorder in suicide attempters. Robins et al. (1959) studied a consecutive sample of individuals who committed suicide in the St. Louis area and found 94% could be given a psychiatric diagnosis (affective disorder 47%, alcoholism 25%, organic brain syndrome 4%, schizophrenia 2%). Likewise, Barraclough et al. (1974) in 100 consecutive suicides in Great Britain found that 93% of the victims had a mental disorder (70% depression, 15% alcoholism).

Dingman and McGlashan (1988), in a 15-year follow-up of severely ill inpatients who had made a serious suicide threat or attempt before admission, wanted to ascertain whether there were characteristics that discriminated those who committed suicide from those who did not. The results demonstrated that patients who committed suicide were more likely to be male, to have a DSM-III (American Psychiatric Association 1980) Axis I diagnosis, and to be discharged against medical advice. Those alive at follow-up were more likely to have borderline personality disorder and to be female, impulsive, and self-mutilating; their postdischarge course was healthier. Of the 403 total sample followed up, 15 patients ultimately killed themselves; of the latter, 22% were schizophrenic, 36% schizoaffective, 5% bipolar, and 43% unipolar.

In a follow-up study of adult suicide attempters, Stone (1989) examined the records of 49 completed suicides from a group of 500 patients hospitalized at New York State Psychiatric Institute. According to diagnoses among the 49 suicides, 9.5% of the schizophrenic group, 23% of the schizoaffective group, 10% of the bipolar group, and 8.9% of the borderline patients had committed suicide. In those borderline patients meeting DSM-III criteria, self-damaging acts, impulsivity, and inordinate anger were associated with heightened suicidality. J. S. Jones et al. (1990) found that 75%–90% of schizophrenic patients who kill themselves are male and under age 45 years; schizophrenic patients who commit suicide typically have severe, chronic, relapsing illness with many exacerbations and hospitalizations. The majority of suicides occurred within the first 10 years after diagnosis.

In both the Stone (1989) and the Dingman and McGlashan (1988) studies, patients with schizoaffective disorder constituted the most suicide-prone group. Of the 49 suicides in Stone's (1989) study, 4 were bipolar. The group size is too small about which to make valid inferences, but he noted that the relationship to violence (jumping, shooting, hanging) was striking. In that study, 6 (12%) of the suicides had at least one first-degree relative with major depressive illness, and 3 had experienced the suicide of one or more of these close relatives. Gunderson (1984) reported that 75% of a sample of borderline inpatients had made at least one suicide gesture. The overall estimate of borderline patients who eventually kill themselves was 10%.

Comorbidity increases suicidal risk. Stone (1989) found that completed suicide was particularly high in male borderline patients meeting DSM-III criteria who also had a major affective disorder (17.9%). Fyer et al. (1988) found that the combination of borderline personality disorder and affective disorder carries a high risk for suicidal behavior particularly when combined with substance abuse.

As in adult suicide attempters there seems to be a high prevalence of psychiatric disorder in adolescent suicide attempters. Weissman (1974) described the typical adolescent at risk for suicide as a male between ages 15 and 19, who had either an affective disorder or schizophrenia, who had a history of behavior problems (conduct disorder, substance abuse, or alcohol), and who exhibited frequent suicidal ideation or suicidal behavior. Ambrosini et al. (1984) observed that the prevalence of major depressive disorder increased up to 80% in children and adolescents who had made serious suicide attempts. They noted the strong association between suicide and 1) depressive disorder and 2) chronic alcoholism. Carlson and Cantwell (1982) noted that 83% of a severely suicidal group of inpatient adolescents also were diagnosed with DSM-III criteria for major depression. Likewise 75% of the severely suicidal group had families with a history of depression or alcoholism. Pfeffer et al. (1988) also found that an analysis of the records of 200 consecutively admitted adolescent psychiatric inpatients revealed that 34% of the patients had made at least one suicide attempt (major depressive and alcohol abuse disorders being the chief diagnoses). Significant predictors of suicidal behavior were alcohol abuse, past suicidal behavior, depression, and aggressive behavior.

With respect to aggression and violence, it has been estimated that 10%–20% of suicidal people have histories of violence, and 30% of violent persons have histories of suicidal behavior (Plutchik and van Praag 1990). A psychological autopsy study of young completed suicides found that almost one-half had histories of aggressive and antisocial behavior, a much higher rate than found in older age groups (Gould et al. 1990). Even in patients who have not acted out violently, overt expression of rage and hostility is more common in depressed patients who are suicidal than in those who are not (Weissman et al. 1973).

Borderline personality disorder is often found concurrent with other disorders; data suggest that its comorbidity with affective disorder and substance abuse increases the lethality and frequency of suicide attempts. Friedman et al. (1982) found that among 76 adolescent inpatients, those who carried an Axis I diagnosis (major affective disorder) as well as Axis II (borderline personality disorder) made more lethal and more frequent attempts than those with only one diagnosis.

In Stone's (1992) sample, of the nine adolescent suicides, five were borderline (all satisfying DSM-III criteria), four presented with a psychosis (manic depressive in one case), and the other three were schizoaffective. Life events such as loss of a caretaker or traumatic experiences often figured importantly as precipitants or background characteristics in the lives of eventual suicides. Traumatic events within the family tend to be more pathogenic in this regard than those external to it; those of particular significance include incest (especially transgenerational: father-daughter or uncle-niece), physical brutality on the part of a parent, or intense verbal humiliation by close family members.

Brent et al. (1988) found four risk factors more prevalent (81.9%) among adolescent suicide victims when compared with those of a group at high risk for suicide: 1) diagnosis of bipolar disorder, 2) affective disorder with comorbidity, 3) lack of previous mental health treatment, and 4) availability of firearms in the homes. Shaffer and Hicks' view (1992) is that conduct disorder leads to antisocial behaviors—drug and alcohol abuse—which subsequently lead to extreme variation in mood, especially depression. Thus a history of conduct disorder in childhood may be predictive of drug abuse, alcoholism, depression, and suicide.

Psychological research. The relationship between stress and suicidal behavior has been considered for years. A. R. Rich and Bonner (1987) have proposed a transactional stress-vulnerability model of suicidal ideation and behavior that proposes that social-emotional alienation, cognitive distortions and inadequate adaptive abilities provide a predispositional base for suicidal behavior. In a retrospective study of college students, the authors found that subjects who scored high in suicidal ideation and behavior were more socially alienated and exhibited more cognitive rigidity and fewer adaptive mechanisms for coping than a nonsuicide comparison group.

The cognitive model of depression and suicidal ideation, conceptualized by Beck (1976) proposes that the patients' personalized and subjective interpretations, expectations, and basic assumptions cause unpleasant emotional states, undesirable behaviors, and other evidences of psychological distress (Bedrosian and Epstein 1984). According to Beck, the "cognitive triad" is the hallmark of the depressed patients' thinking: negative views of the self, the world, and the future. When an individual is deeply depressed, the events in his or her world are perceived in the bleakest possible light. If life is perceived as worthless and there is no meaning to life, despair and hopelessness may lead to contemplation of suicide.

Patsiokas et al. (1979) described a particular personality characteristic of suicidal adults—*cognitive inflexibility*. This term implies a lack of divergent as opposed to convergent thinking, an inability to use innovative ways to solve problems and think in creative and imaginative ways, and to develop alternate strategies when confronted by life stress. Neuringer (1964) believed the suicidal individual can often find no solution to life's problems other than death. Orbach et al. (1987) also studied the relation between some aspects of cognitive inflexibility and suicidal behavior. A group of 27 suicidal children (15 boys and 12 girls, ages 6 to 12 years) was compared with chronically ill and healthy matched control subjects. All were presented with the Suicidal Tendencies Test (developed by Orbach and colleagues [1983]), which measured attitudes toward life and death. The results demonstrated how suicidal children tend to be unable to produce alternative attitudes toward life and death compared with chronically ill or healthy children.

More research has been done in cognitive aspects of suicidal thinking and behavior in adults than in children and adolescents. Dyer and Kreitman (1984), studying adult populations, found that hopelessness was a better predictor of future suicidal behavior than depression. Hopelessness as measured by the Beck Hopelessness Inventory (Beck et al. 1974) was taught to predict future suicide attempts better than either depression or suicidal intent (Beck et al. 1985). Kasdin et al. (1983), in studying similar phenomena in child psychiatric inpatients, found that hopelessness was associated with low self-esteem; they inferred that depressed children also have a negative view of the self, the world, and the future. In attempting to replicate those findings, Asarnow et al. (1987) evaluated factors associated with depression and suicidal behavior in school-age and preadolescent child psychiatric inpatients. They found that depressed children (not necessarily suicidal) did have negative self-perceptions and world views. What differentiated the children with suicidal behavior from children without that behavior was a tendency to perceive their families as low in control and cohesiveness and high in conflict. These children also demonstrated significantly fewer cognitive strategies for coping with stressful life events than nonsuicidal children. Asarnow and Carlson (1988) presented supportive findings. Although actual family stress is a powerful influence on children's behavior, the youngster's perception of the nature and degree of family stress is important in itself. Researchers found strong support (88% accuracy rate) for a link between suicide attempts in children and perceptions of low family support.

Rotheram-Borus and Trautman (1988), however, using the Beck Depression Inventory and Beck Hopelessness Inventory studied a group of minority female adolescents who had attempted suicide. They found that the group did not appear more hopeless than a control group of girls with psychiatric disturbance who had not attempted suicide and felt hopelessness per se was not an indicator of suicidality in minority adolescent girls as it seems to be in adult populations.

Although these studies are preliminary, they are important in explaining the relationships between negative cognitive thinking (inflexibility) and suicidal thinking and behavior. Such research is necessary in planning for successful programs for suicide prevention and intervention.

The puzzle of suicide in general and of adolescent suicide in particular has been enlightened somewhat by the many areas of research into the problem. The various research approaches have provided some knowledge that has not been available previously (most notably that the majority of persons who complete suicide also have Axis I DSM-III-R [American Psychiatric Association 1987] diagnoses). Furthermore, a general consensus exists about some of the more severe risk factors for adolescent suicide. There is growing evidence that genetic and other biological factors play some role in some cases and there are some hints of what some of the biological factors may be. In addition, research corroborates what would otherwise be common-sense knowledge: suicidal children and adolescents think differently than do their nonsuicidal peers.

However, the current state of research does not answer many of the definitive, clinically necessary questions. There is not enough research on the distinctive and specific issues of adolescent suicide. There are contradictory studies in each area of research, and, unfortunately, the committee believes there is not enough knowledge yet to resolve most of the apparent contradictions. Most importantly, there is no answer in hard research to the essential question of what distinguishes those who do fulfill most of the presently understood criteria—those demographically most vulnerable, those who demonstrate many of the risk factors, those who show genetic and biological factors conducive to suicide, those with ominous psychiatric diagnoses, and those who think in dangerously different ways—who do seriously attempt or complete suicide from those with the same characteristics who do not.

It is possible that hard, numbers-oriented research will not provide those answers. It does provide invaluable help for clinical identification of a significant proportion of high-risk adolescents and suggests relevant directions to explore in trying to plan intervention and treatment. However, the individual differences between those who are versus those who are not ultimately suicidal are probably just that: individual. The answers probably lie in unique developmental differences and in specific individual and familial psychodynamic differences that interact with the various risk vulnerabilities (as previously discussed in Chapter 2) in a way that leads to the probability of a fatal outcome.

4

Psychodynamics and Psychopathology Associated With Suicide

The previous chapters have highlighted numerous factors associated with suicide. Cultural, socioeconomic, biological, familial, peer-related, and individual psychological concerns play different roles in suicide depending on the case. Countering the forces that may lead an adolescent to contemplate or attempt suicide are parallel forces in each of the mentioned areas that protect the adolescent from considering such a solution. In this respect, the choice of suicide is not unlike other symptom choices. In the highest crime neighborhoods, most families manage to escape a pattern of delinquency. In chaotic families, one or more children may become achievers. It is apparent that built-in strengths can serve as powerful bulwarks against pressures toward maladaptive behavior. The clinical assessment of suicide potential must address both the propensity for and the strengths against acting self-destructively.

Happy persons do not contemplate suicide. At the same time, unhappiness does not lead inexorably to a suicide wish. We must explore the question of what kind (or degree) of unhappiness or mental disturbance results in suicidal ideation or intent.

The natural reaction to a suicide attempt or completed suicide is to wonder about what immediate stresses might have precipitated the behavior. Yet there is no single event or stimulus that can be considered a necessary and sufficient explanation for the suicidal act. Nor is it possible to identify a unique combination of circumstances that regularly lead to it. Analysis of individual cases reveals a complex mixture of current and historical predisposing factors, of extrinsic and intrinsic stressors, and of specific triggering events.

Early biological and environmental influences determine degrees of vulnerability. Subsequent incursions on the normal process of development may reinforce that vulnerability. By adolescence a youth could be a serious suicide risk. How successfully the tasks of adolescence are then negotiated can be an additional determinant. The extent to which the adolescent can cope successfully with adversity or failure and the availability of real alternatives are important because suicidal adolescents often feel trapped. Finally, the precipitating event may be experienced as an intolerable or irreversible stress that clinches the decision.

In the final analysis, one is dealing with a state of mind, a kind of psychological readiness for self-destruction that sets the suicidal adolescent apart from his or her peers. The willingness to end one's life often suggests that either the value placed on life or the belief that one can reap the rewards it may offer has been seriously compromised. Possibly, in the adolescent's fantasies, death would provide preferable rewards.

Psychodynamic Factors

Hendin (1991) considers psychodynamics as dealing with recurrent conflict patterns and the quality of interpersonal relations—essentially the inner meanings of actions, experiences, and thoughts. He considers the affective states in which suicide is attempted or completed to be rage, guilt, hopelessness, despair, and desperation.

In the genesis of such affects, there are usually important contributing factors in the quality of the parent-child relationship. The child's sense of worth, barring some physical or neurological handicap, is first laid down early in life prior to the school years, mainly from what has been communicated by the parents. Whether life is meaningful and its struggles worth the effort are beliefs first acquired in one's home. The child's sense of competence, established by means of academic, athletic, artistic, social, or other achievement, begins prior to the school years. Both the sense of worth and the feeling of competence are attributes basic to normal growth and development. They appear to be particularly damaged in the suicidal youth.

The crucial contribution of the parents is their responsiveness, or lack of it, to the developing child and adolescent. In one typical scenario, the home is an unhappy place in which the youth feels unloved and his or her needs are not responded to in an appropriately empathic manner. A mother may convey to her son that her depression is his responsibility, he is useless, he contributes nothing to her happiness, and he is a burden. Because of her depression she portrays the world as a miserable place and is helpless to alter her own lot. The boy's father, a possible source of a corrective experience, may passively or actively reinforce these perceptions. The result is various degrees of purposelessness, worthlessness, and impotence. Even in suicides that appear to be the direct consequence of losses or traumatic events in the immediate life experience of the adolescent, pathogenic familial factors appear to play a definitive role in the adolescent's succumbing to rather than surmounting the trauma.

The experiences in a child's or adolescent's life are perceived and interpreted in part according to the limitations of the youngster's cognitive developmental stage. They are also colored by the stage of psychosexual development at which they occur and the drives and needs characteristic of that stage. Out of the experiences, together with the twists put on them through the filter of the child's immature cognitive and psychological capacities, the youngster evolves the private and idiosyncratic meanings he or she assigns to the important events and people in his or her life, and to his or her own life as well. They become the personal themes and myths by which life is lived. These meanings, or psychodynamics, along with the associated emotions, shape the ways in which he or she perceives new events and the future in general. They come to motivate behavior and relationships. In the cases of early pathogenic influences so frequently found in suicidal adolescents, these meanings and motivations are usually distorted, maladaptive, even bizarre.

The adolescent who attempts suicide is usually caught up in an inner web of fantasies and beliefs that seem to give some logical meaning and purpose to the wish for death. Although these motifs may not be as crucial as some risk factors in assessing immediate suicidality, they clarify important aspects of the person's plan, his or her appreciation of death, and his or her relationships with the important people in his or her life. The person's ability to distinguish fantasy from reality may indeed make these private myths crucial in assessing suicidality because the capacity to test reality may make the difference between fantasied action and tangible lethal behavior.

Harold, a 17-year-old boy, had been referred for therapy when he was 12, following the death of his mother, and had been seen weekly since that time. His family life was disorganized and abusive. Over the years since her death, he has had recurrent suicidal ideation motivated primarily by the fantasy of reunion with his mother after death, on which he elaborates in poetry and song lyrics. His suicidality has at times been serious enough that he has thought out plans and means, but he has never actively attempted it. While in the throes of relentless thoughts of being unable to secure an unattainable love object (he had also recently been spurned by a girlfriend), he read for the first time von Goethe's *The Sorrows of Young Werther and Novella* (1990). He readily identified, if not merged, with Werther whose suicide was also rationalized by the fantasy of reunion after death.

This adolescent's suicidality is clearly motivated by a maladaptive fantasy developed after his mother's death. A variety of other psychodynamic themes has emerged through work with other patients. These meanings are not always conscious, and the youngster may not be able to formulate them in response to questions; they may become clear only through dreams or free associations.

Hendin (1991) suggests that all psychodynamic meanings of suicide can be conceptualized as responses to loss, separation, or abandonment. We would add that these traumas may be real or fantasied, may be past, current, or anticipated, and that the core meaning of every suicide attempt is to assert some control over situations that the adolescent considers intolerable, and before which he or she feels helpless to influence in a more rational, less dramatic manner. The ways in which suicidal adolescents imagine their deaths will cope somehow with the perceived unbearable situation are almost infinitely variable.

Reunion after death, as in the vignette above, is a frequent theme in which magical control over loss is sought, and as discussed in Chapter 2, is a frequent motive in Danish suicides. A related dynamic is the fantasy that life is reversible or repeatable, that one can be reborn. The fantasy may be that, "After I die, I can start life over and get a fresh start," or "I can be a child again, have an all-good, all-loving mother and be happy."

Suicide may be an effort to control and alleviate guilt through self-punishment and atonement. Sexual guilt is still an important dynamic, but it may easily be overlooked in an era when sexual permissiveness is widely assumed to be the norm among adolescents. It still can occur in grossly excessive degrees: "If I kill myself, then God and mother will forgive me for my promiscuity," or "I can't stand this dirty body, these filthy feelings and thoughts; after I die I'll be rid of them and be innocent again." More common currently is guilt over failure to live up to parental or societal expectations that have come to form one's own punitive ego-ideal as in many Japanese youth suicides: "If I kill myself, I will atone for losing my scholarship," or "My death is the only way to save my family's honor since I've gotten illegitimately pregnant."

The desire for revenge and retaliation is a powerful suicide motivator. It is often conscious as in, "After I'm gone, you'll be sorry for how you treated me and my suicide will haunt you the rest of your life," or "You've been so mean and neglectful, now you'll have to think of me; maybe you'll appreciate how good I've been and how much I loved you." Often the vengeful motive is less conscious, and a suicide that appears to be an escape from an abusive or overdemanding and over-controlling parental environment also includes the magical belief that the internalized hated other will also be destroyed: "When I kill myself I'll be free of your mistreatment and you'll be gone too; I've always wished you were dead, and you'll never be able to hurt me again."

In a reversal of or in combination with a vengeful motive, youngsters are sometimes acting out death wishes by parents (or perhaps others) toward themselves. Such death wishes may be unconsciously or overtly conveyed and unconsciously or consciously perceived. These devastating feelings of rejection seem controllable only through death. "I know you don't want me; you and everyone else will be better off when I'm gone. Maybe you'll be sorry too." Similarly, youngsters who come to feel themselves to be worthless or bad may believe that they deserve to be dead and that death is an appropriate punishment for them. Their suicide then becomes self-fulfilling of their expectation.

Adolescents may try to control a dysfunctional or disintegrating family system by becoming a suicidal scapegoat, a rallying point for the family. This may be an unconscious dynamic covered over by the consciously perceived, out-of-control distress the youngster feels. If the attempt fails, this maneuver can at times be successful if competent and family-oriented emergency and long-term intervention is mobilized.

Although magical or realistic control over catastrophe is a meaning in all suicidal dynamics, at times it becomes the most overt and prominent. When death actually threatens an adolescent as in an apparently incurable illness, in suicide the person controls the time of death rather than being a helpless victim of disease progression. A loss that feels tantamount to death may be anticipated and the adolescent may need to demonstrate control over the fear of loss (death): "I'm not afraid to be hurt; I'm not afraid to be on my own and alone. I might as well be dead and I'm not even afraid of death."

The dynamic motivations of most suicide attempts begin in early, primitive developmental stages when there is no clear separation between self and other. There is usually the fantasy that the self-destructive act will influence or affect some other as though that other is still a part of, inseparable from, the self. That these fantasies live on in suicidal adolescents (as well as in suicidal adults) indicates that the adolescent is not functioning beyond that primitive stage. However, there is an intermixture of reality, particularly in revenge and escape suicides, of which the adolescent may be acutely aware and may give him or her great manipulative power. Suicide may not affect the hated other in the magical ways characteristic of the primitive fantasies, but adolescents can inflict overwhelming pain and remorse that the youngster somehow fantasizes he or she will witness and gloat over. Also, many adolescents have real and devastating conditions from which to escape.

Although these fantasies and personal myths are often elaborated toward significant others such as parents, friends, or lovers, and indeed may always originate with parents, they will often appear in the clinical situations and interfere with and contaminate the relationship that is meant to save the adolescent—especially because it is the relationship with the therapist that helps the patient stay alive.

The reality of the escape motive in many suicide attempts may correspond to the dreadful reality of some adolescents' lives and raises the question of suicide that may not reflect intrapsychic pathology or the overriding psychopathology of major psychiatric illness. Escape suicide often bespeaks the adolescent's cognitive and psychological immaturity in that he or she cannot grasp and use more appropriate alternatives. It may be that limited cognitive style (see Chapter 3) limits options. Inappropriate primitive fantasies derived from parental pathogenicity may weaken the adolescent's ability to value known and available alternatives.

However, there can be genuinely overwhelming conditions in many adolescents' lives. The severely and chronically sexually and physically abused girl may not know of remedial alternatives or may live where they are not available to her. The boy dying of AIDS may know with certainty the misery of the most terminal stages and appropriately recognize the unlikelihood of some medical miracle coming along to cure and reverse his condition at the stage at which he finds himself. It seems not necessary always to insist on some individual psychopathology over and above such unacceptable life circumstances. Altruistic suicide, although not a form of escape, also may not inevitably argue psychopathology.

Some may insist that these kinds of suicide might be understandable in adulthood or old age, but not in adolescence when formal thinking is often not fully established, when the meaning and process of death may not be understood, and when the adolescent still struggles to establish an identity and a sense of self. Whether or not self-destruction is justified in these situations or for these reasons is a question the individual must ask about his or her life.

The philosophical issue of existential suicide extends beyond such palpable catastrophes. Even if one grants some validity to the position in general—difficult to negate *in toto*—its applicability to adolescence is in most instances debatable at least.

Existential philosophers believe that human beings have a right to die, a right to choose when to die, and a right to choose the method by which to die; man's principal life task is to respond to and deal with the lack of meaning, the absurdity, and the despair in life (Schneidman 1979). Life is a struggle and a painful one and only death can end the problem of being human. Anything short of suicide is an inadequate adaptation to the major problem of life—life itself. Only death solves life.

The existentialist validates his or her position by asking us to consider what life would be like if all suicides would be prevented and eliminated. "The optimum suicide rate is not zero. . . . We could easily have a zero suicide rate, but I suspect none of us would want to live in such a world. Many things are far worse than suicide" (Maris 1989, p. 456). It is death and the possibility of suicide that gives meaning to life (Maris 1989).

A consideration of philosophical or existential suicide has its place in general discussion of suicide, especially adult suicide. It is, however, irrelevant to an understanding of adolescent suicide although one can try to understand the adolescent's viewpoint. The adolescent invests in new idealizations and experiences gradual or precipitous deidealizations that are worked through in acquiring personal ideals and value systems. Many adolescents are in love with their newfound capacities for philosophizing and may be fascinated with the power they have discovered to cause their own death. This is not truly the existential position of the man or woman who has seen life, who can speak of the absurdity of existence. The adolescent who thinks and speaks in this fashion is working out identity and self issues.

A physician dedicated to relieving pain and helping others achieve health finds the existential position unacceptable because he or she knows that severe depression or a powerful, time-limited impulse will usually abate even without treatment. The responsible physician believes in trying to keep the person alive until the depression lifts or until perspective on the impulse can be gained. A clinical perspective demands an investigation for the underlying psychopathology. Existential suicide implies free choice, a philosophical position that must be considered in accord with the adolescent's level of development. A clinician following the Hippocratic oath would find it difficult to agree that suicide is justified; he or she must always try to prevent it even though friends and family afterward may hold that a person's suicide, including an adolescent's, was reasonable and not pathological.[1] Often, adolescent suicide is idealized in the media, but to the family, friends, and victim, there is nothing ideal. Unfortunately, such media treatment ignores underlying clinical problems.

Psychopathology of Suicidal Behavior in Psychiatric Syndromes

Suicidal behavior occurs in patients with a variety of diagnostic syndromes and illnesses. The existence of a major psychiatric illness or a diagnosable condition does not negate the existence or the significance of internal meanings and psychodynamics related to prior life experiences and which may in part motivate the suicidality or help to determine its nature and timing. In some instances, such as neuroses and character disorders, the same childhood traumata that are the basis of the inner myths and fantasies are those that most significantly cause and determine the nature of the illnesses themselves. In the more severe illnesses such as psychoses (and perhaps others) in which biological or genetic factors may have a causative role independent of life events, psychodynamic meanings still exist but are variously distorted by the illness itself. The individual may imagine traumata that never occurred or exaggerate or distort what negative experiences did occur. The psychotically colored fantasies may still be clinically important in influencing the circumstances and the times when the patient is most at risk,

---

[1]The current situation of physician-assisted suicide to relieve intractable suffering accompanying some imminently fatal illnesses has raised questions that may modify this position.

the form of the suicide attempt, and consequently the nature of therapeutic interventions.

In less severe psychiatric conditions, fantasy can function to absorb aggression and pain from internal and external psychological pressures (Grossman 1991). Neurotic children with mild psychiatric disturbances characterized by anxiety and mild depression (dysthymic disorder) may have suicidal ideas and fantasies that they consider a *possible* solution, not *the* solution. Moreover, this child will be more aware of the repercussions of death to himself or herself and to others. Not infrequently the child will share his or her suicidal ideation with adults.

> A 13-year-old girl was brought to the emergency room one evening because of suicidal ideation. The patient said she had grown up without a father and that her mother had recently remarried. She felt a previously idyllic situation had become stressful. She reported the only reason she had not killed herself was that she had asked her aunt what would happen if a person killed herself and her aunt had responded that the person would go to hell. The patient was willing to contract for her safety and with the support of her family agreed to be seen in the outpatient department.

Youngsters with a dysthymic disorder or a mild depression may have suicidal ideation and make suicidal gestures. At times, suicidal behaviors lie behind the overt reasons that the child is referred for psychiatric evaluation.

> A 16-year-old male was brought to the emergency room by the family in the early evening because of school truancy. During the interview the patient revealed suicidal ideation and an episode the previous week in which he had put his father's loaded gun to his head but had been afraid to pull the trigger. When the patient's father was told of the need for admission, his first response was that things were not really so bad. The father stated he would take his son home and think about the recommendation for hospitalization. When the patient's father was then told that his son had held a loaded gun to his head, the father reluctantly agreed to admission. During the hospitalization the patient revealed that his father had tried to kill himself several years previously.

Posttraumatic stress disorder is often a more severe expression of adjustment reactions and neurotic reactions and represents a high-risk factor for suicide. The patient may be suicidal after witnessing parental suicidality. Thirty children whose parents made a suicide attempt requiring hospitalization reenacted the witnessed suicidal act so dramatically in play and behavior that one could identify the details of their parents' suicide attempts (e.g., stabbing themselves with rubber knives or taking pills). Their cognition also was affected by disruptive thoughts and efforts to deny the experience and they experienced depression and impulsive behavior well into adolescence (Pynoos and Eth 1985).

Even more at risk are adolescents who have made suicide attempts and have ideation associated with violent plans.

Under a combination of stresses and a cultural tradition that premarital sex and abortion are sinful, a 15-year-old female, 4 months pregnant, was seen in the emergency room after an overdose of ibuprofen. After discovering her pregnancy, the patient wished to have an abortion but had been forced by her family to continue the pregnancy. She became depressed and agitated and the family forced her to leave the home. She was taken in by an aunt. The day of the suicide attempt the patient's boyfriend said that he wanted to end their relationship. A fight ensued after which the boyfriend took an overdose of pills and was admitted to the same hospital's intensive care unit. As the patient was not allowed to visit her boyfriend, she subsequently overdosed as well. During the hospitalization, the patient also admitted to thoughts of jumping from a second story window to induce an abortion.

This adolescent's suicidal behaviors were preceded by a number of stressors including pregnancy out of wedlock, prohibition of abortion, parental rejection, and loss of her boyfriend.

Severe risk is presented by adolescents with major affective disorders.

A 17-year-old depressed girl was admitted after an overdose. The patient's family was very upset about the fact that the she was initially admitted to the schizophrenia unit because there were no beds on the adolescent unit. They became so upset about this that they demanded she be discharged. There were three other family members with bipolar disorder and the family and parents complained about their negative past experiences with psychiatrists. The patient was subsequently hospitalized involuntarily. The family then hired a lawyer who had the commitment rescinded. The patient shot and killed herself 2 weeks later.

Patients with severe conduct disorders can present suicidal behaviors that are characterized by aggression, revenge, and retaliation within a context of impulsivity and ingestion of alcohol and drugs.

A 14-year-old female with a lifelong history of family instability was seen in the outpatient clinic for evaluation because of suicidal ideation. The patient reported living with her mother until her mother began a new romantic relationship, and the patient was sent to live with her aunt and uncle in another city. She moved back and forth several times a year. At age 12, she developed a preoccupation with a punk rock star who had killed his girlfriend and then committed suicide. At age 14, she began making suicide gestures with small overdoses and had also begun cutting herself superficially and had one previous hospitalization for an overdose. On the day of the evaluation, the patient was dressed in black-and-white punk attire. She admitted to an ongoing preoccupation with suicide and stated that she viewed suicide as a way of joining her idol. She reported no active suicide plan at the time of the first evaluation session but indicated escalating suicidality during the ensuing sessions. She admitted to sleeping with a knife and to waking during the night to cut her chest, abdomen, and arms. She was hospitalized at that point on a long-term adolescent unit. This patient demonstrates not only a vulnerability to external stressors but also a clear progression from suicidal ideation to suicidal preoccupation to suicidal gestures and finally to suicidal attempts.

Depression and conduct disorders frequently overlap.[2] Depression contributes inconsistently to a suicide attempt and is neither necessary nor sufficient for it (Carlson and Cantwell 1982). Many suicidal youngsters are not overtly depressed but have conduct disorder. Indeed, suicidality scored on the Kiddie-SADS (a childhood version of the Schedule for Affective Disorders and Schizophrenia) were higher in adolescents with conduct disorders than in adolescents with major affective disorders (Apter et al. 1988). In addition to clear-cut diagnostic criteria for unipolar or bipolar depression, all these patients came from severely disturbed living situations that usually activate the suicidal behavior (Carlson and Cantwell 1982) such as overt rejection by parents, incest, violence, divorce, drug abuse, and suicidal behaviors in other members of the family.

Major affective disorders, schizophrenia, or schizoaffective illness present severe risks of suicide, especially for patients with a recent history of bizarre or impulsive suicidal behavior even though they do not appear to be clinically depressed (O. F. Kernberg 1991). Patients with psychotic disorders frequently make attempts or complete suicide without

---

[2] Personality disorders, such as borderline personality disorder, achieve full expression in adulthood. However, features of these disorders may begin to show themselves in adolescence.

having made previous suicidal attempts (Stone 1992). Their behavior can be bizarre, violent, and more lethal because reality testing and judgment are severely curtailed or abolished.

> A 16-year-old girl was hospitalized because of suicidal ideation, gender confusion, social withdrawal, and a recent 20-pound weight loss. She had been hospitalized briefly 1 year earlier after threatening to jump in front of a train. Shy and withdrawn all her life, she became more severely so after her menarche at age 12. She began to develop a delusional system believing herself to have two selves—one female whom she found disgusting and one male self that made her do and say "bad things." On the unit she made no eye contact, dressed in male attire, laughed inappropriately, and showed blunted affect. She displayed suicidal ideation and spoke of feeling unreal for the past 3 years. Although bright academically, she had begun having trouble concentrating on her schoolwork. She became preoccupied with dirt and germs. To avoid feelings of hopelessness she tried to sleep as much as possible yet felt her bed was made of quicksand where she would sink and die. Diagnosed schizoaffective, she did not respond to neuroleptic treatment or antidepressants. One year later she was transferred to another hospital, and 1 month later she took a fatal overdose while on a pass (Stone 1992).

The psychotic patient may seek suicide as a relief for the psychotic experience—be that extreme states of annihilation anxiety, persecution, or extreme hopelessness—as the individual realizes his or her difference from others.

> An autistic adolescent patient had been treated since he was age 5 with intensive psychoeducational and psychotherapeutic approaches. He was improved enough to be able to carry out his bar mitzvah, learn computers, and become a computer instructor in the special summer camp he attended. As he became progressively aware of his differences from his older brother who was a normal young college student and from his gifted sister, he became extremely suicidal. He contemplated his death either by throwing himself off the balcony or by having somebody kill him. This required active intervention by his therapist until he was able to come to grips with his difference. Had it not been for this treatment and finding a more appropriate environmental situation in a protected community he would almost certainly have succeeded in killing himself. Indeed, he had considered a variety of suicidal plans, had set a date for himself, and was preoccupied with finding relief for his pain by "disappearing from the surface of the earth."

Anorexia nervosa involves slow, self-destructive behavior (i.e., self-starvation). At times it may involve psychotic thinking such as the belief that one's self will survive. However, anorexia nervosa and bulimia in general also show an increased incidence of suicide probably because of the concomitant, frequently associated depression.

A 12-year-old girl who came for evaluation and weighed 38 pounds said she was feeling so weak that she was barely able to walk. She was convinced that even if she stopped eating altogether, she would be alive because "just her body would be dead" and not her herself. There was no other indication of psychotic ideation.

The more severe the impairment caused by a psychiatric disorder, the more vulnerable the patient is to the vicissitudes of his or her environment. For example, in periods of change in inpatient or residential settings such as staff turnover or moves to other locations, the high vulnerability of suicidal patients to such changes is often accentuated. All of the predisposing life experiences and the psychodynamic factors triggering suicidal behavior in adolescents are thus much more influential in patients who have a psychiatric disorder.

5

Prevention and Early Intervention With the Suicidal Adolescent

It is useful to consider the identifications of and interventions with respect to suicidal adolescents in three successive categories or levels. First are *primary* or prevention and identification aspects. The *secondary* level is the acute phase intervention with an actively suicidal youngster. The *tertiary* level is the ongoing therapeutic work with the adolescent, the family, or others when there is ongoing suicidal potential but not acute suicidal ideation or plans. The first two of these categories are addressed in this chapter; the issues of ongoing therapeutic approaches will be taken up in Chapter 7.

Primary or Preventive Interventions

Peggy, a 17-year-old female, was referred by her pediatrician to a child psychiatry clinic for evaluation of an eating disorder. She had lost 10 pounds in 2 months and her mother was concerned. Evaluation by her doctor had found no organic cause for her weight loss. At the clinic she stated that she was not trying to lose weight, had begun to sleep poorly about 2 months ago unless she had several beers, and that she and friends "got trashed" on weekends. Her relationship with her parents was poor; she had attempted suicide a year previously with aspirin and was briefly hospitalized. The day before this evaluation she had taken a razor to school to try to cut her wrists, but it was taken away by a friend. She admitted

being depressed and wanting to commit suicide and finally told of discovering that she was pregnant 4 months earlier. Her boyfriend wanted
her to abort, she was ambivalent, and then she miscarried spontaneously
about 2 months after her discovery. After that, "It didn't really matter how
I felt about anything." Peggy's family was found to be chaotic and unable
to provide a safe environment so she was admitted to a psychiatric hospital on the basis of multiple known risk factors.

The most important aspect of any suicide prevention effort is the
early recognition of the adolescent at increased risk for suicide. The
majority of these adolescents do not come to the attention of mental
health professionals before their suicide. Shaffer et al. (in press) showed
that 46% of individuals who completed suicides had a lifetime history
of some form of psychotherapy compared with 20% of matched control
subjects. Of those that completed suicide, 20% had seen a mental health
professional in the 3 months before their suicide compared with 5% of
the control subjects. Hawton and Blackstock (1976) have shown that in
their sample that was not restricted to adolescents, 36% had contacted
their physicians during the week before their suicidal act, and more than
60% had done so in the month beforehand. Sixty-three percent had visited them for a variety of psychiatric and social reasons during the preceding year and had nearly all been prescribed psychotropic drugs,
usually tranquilizers or sedatives. These were commonly the drugs taken
in the acts of self-poisoning. In a study limited to adolescent suicide
attempters, 25% had visited their primary care physician during the week
before their attempt, and 50% had seen their physician in the month
before the attempt (Hawton et al. 1982). This finding underscores the
need to involve and educate family members, pediatricians, and other
primary care physicians as well as the need for teachers and peers to
recognize the high-risk adolescent. A program of basic outreach and
education targeted to the groups of adults mentioned above as well as
toward adolescents could play an important role in the prevention of
adolescent suicide.

Primary approaches to prevention of adolescent suicide would include, but not be necessarily limited to the following:

1. An overarching priority would be the detection and treatment of
    those psychiatric disorders accompanied by high suicidal risk:
    depression, conduct disorders, borderline conditions, and schizo-
    affective disorders. Shaffer et al. (1988) considered that preventive
    strategies are best applied to high-risk groups because most sui-
    cides occur among those with identifiable psychiatric disorders.

2. All threats of suicide, even vague ones voiced to anyone in the adolescent's milieu, should be taken seriously. Such adolescents require immediate psychiatric assessment.

3. Increasing primary physician educational programs would improve their awareness of the warning signs of depression (often masked by acting out and antisocial behaviors in adolescents) and other high suicidal risk psychiatric disorders in adolescents. Programs should stress the frequency with which suicidal adolescents consult their primary care physicians shortly before an attempted or completed suicide. Educational programs should make a special point of dispelling the myth that asking about suicidal intentions will put the idea into the youngster's head and is therefore dangerous. Adolescents usually yearn for someone sharp enough and concerned enough to detect such despair and to bring it into the open so that some help may be made available. Most clinicians are probably not aware of early warning signs that are most likely to manifest themselves to peers, family, or school personnel (see below), but such signs should be included in physician education programs.

. Increasing peer education in the adolescent population is important. This should be done through schools, churches, neighborhood and other social and sports organizations, and the media (especially television). It should include publication and discussion of warning signs and risk factors and advice on the actions to take and options available if one suspects one has a suicidal or depressed friend.

Some schools have begun to implement suicide education programs, en despite resistance from some school personnel. Such programs tend promote knowledge of risk factors, foster beneficial attitudes toward icidal adolescents, and encourage appropriate responses to suicidal essages from peers. Medically technical risk factors such as those associated with serious psychiatric illness are less known and probably s useful to an at-risk adolescent's peers. However, the more obvious, rden variety of signs are those that peers or nonprofessional adult sociates of a teenager are in the best position to detect.

The most ominous warning signs are probably best known: talking peatedly about one's own death, talking of reunions with lost important persons, and giving away prized possessions. Early and more nonecific signs may include

*   Withdrawal from peers and significant others;
*   Poor coping and problem-solving skills in the face of repeated problems;

- Recent social stresses;
- Self-destructive behaviors such as risk-taking; automobile and other accidents; drug and alcohol use; sexual promiscuity; or eating disorders; and
- Recent environmental stresses such as problems at school or home, loss of a job, loss of a friend or girlfriend or boyfriend, or impending notification of parents of poor school or job performance.

Although some of the danger signals may seem obvious, Norton et al. (1989) found that a substantial number of adolescents do not recognize in their peers common signs such as an expressed desire to die, a worried appearance, past or present suicidal gestures or threats, the breakup of a relationship, and school problems. Nearly half of the adolescents questioned believed that such behaviors were unlikely to be related to suicide. In addition, attitudes toward suicidal peers were shown to be generally negative. Norton et al. found that teenagers were poorly prepared to respond appropriately to suicidal messages from a peer, and the more negative attitudes were naturally associated with less ability to respond appropriately. Any awareness of such negativism would discourage a youngster from confiding in his or her associates and increase the sense of isolation—a known risk factor. All of these circumstances imply that a significant number of suicidal adolescents remain unidentified by their peers and are then perhaps more likely to go on to attempt suicide.

A knowledgeable adolescent who suspects that a friend is in danger should be helped to do all he or she can to persuade that friend to talk with a responsible adult. Kalafat and Elias (1992) studied a sample of 325 suburban high school students and their knowledge of suicidal peers, whether they had ever talked to a suicidal peer, and if so, what they actually did in that situation. Ninety-seven students reported having talked with a peer who was considering suicide. Of these, 63% talked with their peer about his or her actions, 24.7% told an adult, and 12% did nothing. Ninth graders were significantly more likely to do nothing compared with eleventh graders.

The adult ultimately involved must also be knowledgeable enough to take the danger signs seriously and respond with appropriate actions. One of the most difficult goals in peer education is to convince the adolescent whose friend refuses that advice to bring these concerns to a responsible adult. They have often been "sworn" to secrecy by the troubled friend, and they are often, if not usually, too immature and too self-concerned with regard to how they may look to their peers to recognize that the seeming betrayal of an inappropriately demanded seal of confidence is a minor—much less an honorable—consequence compared with a peer's potential death. Even in the absence of a specific demand for secrecy, adolescents are busy separating psychologically from parents and adults and arrogating for themselves (generally prematurely) an adult capacity to run their own lives and problems. Peers and friends may believe they can handle their friend's distress adequately themselves. Even when they feel frightened and do not know what to do, there may still be great developmental hesitancy to trust an adult with an admission of helplessness—a delay that can risk the suicidal adolescent's life.

Peck (1985) outlined some of the systematic attempts to combine intervention with prevention among young people in school. Along with similar emphasis on teaching the youngster the need to break the secrecy pattern, he emphasizes discussion groups relating to issues of life, death, loss, depression, and suicide; programs designed to teach students how to help one another; and seminars with staff members and parents with the goals of increasing their awareness of suicide risk factors and enhancing communication skills.

Because peers are often the first to be able to detect a friend's suicidality and because the normally closed nature of teenage social groups adds its own impediments to communication with adults, intense and effective peer education about suicide should have a high priority among primary preventive measures.

5. *Increasing family and general adult education:* Families need to understand the role of family dynamics and of recent family turmoil in precipitating suicidal behavior. Adults in general need a greater consciousness of what to be alert to in adolescents they are involved with and a greater preparedness to respond appropriately when a teen at risk comes to their attention. Rightly or wrongly, teens often blame parents and other family members for their despair; because of this sometimes unfair perception, family members may be the last people the suicidal adolescent would turn to, and if they are sound enough to want adult assistance, it often will be from a person not involved with family.

6. *Reducing the availability of the means of suicide:* Essentially, the effectiveness of this relates chiefly to impulsive suicide; those who carefully plan suicide can always find means. In general, this could involve limiting the availability of dangerous medications and firearms. In the former instance, some have suggested limiting the quantity of over-the-counter medications adolescents can buy or

promoting more widespread use of individual tablet packaging to lessen the likelihood of suddenly grabbing a handful of pills. Regarding firearms, unavailability could inhibit the impulsive use of a highly lethal means, but the limitation of this approach to overall suicide prevalence has already been mentioned. When an individual youngster is known or thought to be acutely suicidal, specific measures of hiding, locking away, or disposing of such means may need to be an immediate emergency measure in their home or other environment.

7. *Making available 24-hour suicide hot lines*: Their efficacy has been questioned by some research groups, whereas others consider that they provide a worthwhile service and a valuable link to available services for adolescents in crisis (although it must be noted that some students report feeling worse after contact with a hot line responder). Hot lines are apparently used more often by females than males. The gender of the responder may play a role in efficacy, opposite-sex responders being perceived as more helpful. Ideally, the volunteers are supervised by mental health professionals. Parents or other authorities should be contacted with or without permission in any perceived emergency or acute need. These hot line programs could be enhanced if 1) they were more aggressively advertised among high-risk groups, 2) there was effective training of the staff for eliciting adequate history and identification and for offering the most helpful and empathic responses, and 3) the staff at the hot line were taught that there is greater compliance by the troubled teenager with referral when the responder makes the referral appointment himself or herself and then follows up later with the youngster to learn if the appointment has been kept.

8. *Organizing programs that involve the media in increasing the awareness* of those who decide the policy of what is printed, aired, or shown both to the suicidogenic effects of highly publicized suicides and also to the great suicide prevention potential of balancing or accompanying such publicity with factual education about suicide. Existing research supports the position that media coverage (both television and newspaper) of real suicides causes an increase in imitative suicides (L. Davidson and Gould 1991); there is little research, and data are contradictory, regarding the presentation of fictional suicide stories. Media reports often idealize or glorify suicidal adolescents. The reports associate suicide with existential social and political stresses but neglect to report that such "causes"

seldom precipitate suicide except in the context of serious psychiatric illness and often gloss over the enormous individual and interpersonal tragedy of the death. Publicized reports of the suicide of well-known, popular personalities also are followed causally by an increased suicide incidence.

It is probably wishful and not even rational thinking to hope that the media as a whole would eschew coverage of suicides to potentially save lives. Suicides are news items of drama and broad community interest, and the media will appropriately report news. However, the manner of the reporting and the additional information included may be influenced by educational programs. It is crucial to highlight suicide as a sign of psychiatric disturbance and to discourage the hero image of the misunderstood youth as the victim of the ills of society. Gould (1992) recommended an ongoing dialogue between the media and mental health organizations to support such a change in presentation, to discourage massive doses of coverage, and to encourage the simultaneous publication of the telephone numbers of clinics and hot lines. We recommend the inclusion of a warning, such as the Surgeon General's warning on cigarette packages, of a brief but prominent list of risk factors and warning signs to educate readers, listeners, and viewers.

Although this report recommends school-based peer education as part of an effort to identify adolescents at risk and to help prevent suicide—ignorance never helps any effort—the value of such programs has been questioned. The research of Shaffer et al. (1988) into the efficacy of some suicide prevention programs found no evidence that actual suicide or suicide attempt rates were reduced by the preventive measures studied. They questioned whether such school programs actually increase suicidal risk. They suggested that a program may be effective if it were focused on the high risk adolescents (Shaffer et al. 1988). In addition, because it is known that information can be suggestive, particularly with adolescents, the manner and context of providing information is an important issue and a reason for urging proper training to those who give this information to adolescents.

The nature of the program also is crucial. Is the program under the management of an "outside" team of suicide-researchers where there may be little or no relationship with the school mental health personnel or is the program conceived and conducted by known school mental health workers or those already involved in health classes and ongoing student groups? To answer some of these questions, the Ottawa Board of Education developed a comprehensive school-based suicide prevention and early intervention program called Skills for Living which was then evaluated. The comprehensive model was composed of

- *Prevention* (sensitization of school personnel, sensitization of parents, teacher training, and curriculum delivery);
- *Intervention policy and procedure* (identification of adolescents at risk and clinical follow-up by school personnel and community mental health professionals); and
- *Postvention* (tragic events school-based response team).

The curriculum was taught by familiar teachers leading small groups in sessions lasting 50 minutes. A matched sample of children in schools not participating in the study was tested pre- and postprogram along with the study children. An initial screening questionnaire indicated that 19% of the students were found to need a second clinical screening. Of those selected for the second screening 61% were judged to be at high suicidal risk; thus the behavior of selected students could be monitored. Results from the study demonstrated that the prevention program did not increase or reduce suicidal behaviors in general, but that the high risk students could be closely monitored in the context of the prevention program (S. Davidson et al. 1990). The opinion of the GAP Committee on Adolescence is that schools can offer a suicide prevention program within the framework of a positive mental health climate. Berkovitz (1985) has suggested five necessary elements to ensure the successful functioning of a suicide prevention program:

1. A positive mental health atmosphere in the individual school and district;
2. An adequate psychological services staff;
3. A suicide prevention program;
4. Adequate health services for suicide intervention; and
5. A suicide postvention program for helping the friends and staff who survive the suicide.

In trying to understand the somewhat confusing and even contradictory material regarding the efficacy of school-based suicide prevention programs, one must recognize the great difficulty in evaluating the programs and their effectiveness. The rarity of adolescent suicide (even though it is a serious problem) makes statistical comparisons difficult. Because only about 1 of 10,000 adolescents commit suicide per year, it would be nearly impossible to collect a large enough number of cases exposed to such programs versus cases not so exposed to permit comparison. In the study of Shaffer et al. (1988), the only research conducted by that team consisted of comparing student knowledge and attitudes with and without and before and after exposure to three different prevention programs; they found no statistical differences. However, they note that attitudes may not always predict behavior when faced with an emergency. The most serious problem in evaluating efficacy is that various programs differ so widely in content, format, length of exposure, and in the leaders that conducted them that they cannot be equated or their effects compared with suicidality in students from schools without prevention programs. Although more studies of specific prevention programs for targeted groups are imperative, we believe now that the school atmosphere should reflect the approaches outlined in this report.

Secondary or Acute Intervention

Knowledge of factors and danger signals with regard to adolescent suicidality, which we have detailed, can alert those who may thereby recognize a potentially or actively suicidal adolescent and get the youngster to professional help. In this section, the focus is on how the professional elicits the crucial information and gathers the data necessary for a medical disposition for a specific adolescent. Suicidal behavior constitutes a medical emergency and an evaluation should be done as soon as possible. The usual setting is the emergency room of a general hospital, although a private psychiatrist may be the initial evaluator. Regardless of who the first evaluator may be, if suicidality is recognized, the definitive evaluation must be by a psychiatrist.

Whenever possible, the evaluator should be a psychiatrist trained in management of emergency, life-threatening situations. A background in child and adolescent evaluation and treatment, together with skill in eliciting relevant information not only from adolescent patients but also from their families and friends, is crucial.[1] In situations where a psychiatrist with these qualifications is not immediately available on site, consultation with a qualified psychiatrist should be available at all times. In teaching hospitals, where the initial evaluator in the emergency room

---

[1]There are many professionally "vacant" rural areas in the world, even in the United States, such as in large areas of Alaska where such ideal recommendations are impossible to implement. Such conditions present special problems that are beyond the scope of this report.

is a resident, it is of utmost importance that the resident have a senior child or adolescent psychiatrist or one experienced with adolescent patients available at all times for consultation; this is crucial both for the patient's welfare and for the resident's training. The on-site evaluator should be specifically trained to ask questions about suicidal ideation and previous attempts, about specific suicide plans, and about family history of suicidal behavior. The evaluating physician must be empathic and firmly dedicated to the affirmation of life; ambivalent feelings about the value of living or dialogues about the meaning of life have no place in the evaluation of suicidal adolescents. Personal beliefs and emotional responses, often unconscious, are seldom more powerfully present than with a suicidal child or adolescent.

Rarely, a suicidal adolescent will come in alone; usually one or more friends or a family member will accompany the youngster. Proper evaluation involves not only the youngster, but family and friends as well, and the most significant persons must be contacted and interviewed if they are not initially present.

Evaluation of the Adolescent

In assessing the suicidal adolescent, if there was an attempt, the details of the attempt must be explored. How lethal was the attempt in terms of method (10 aspirin versus jumping from a high place)? What was the youngster's perception of the lethality? A teenager who believes that 10 aspirin are a fatal dose is as dangerously suicidal as one who shoots himself or herself but misses a vital organ. Was the act done impulsively, or premeditated over days or weeks (taking a handful of whatever was available in the medicine cabinet versus carefully collecting an amount of something thought sure to be deadly)? What does the adolescent say about the attempt? Was there a suicide note? Was there a probability of discovery, or was the attempt made in isolation with intervention unlikely? Was the patient under the influence of alcohol or other drugs at the time of the attempt? What are the adolescent's fantasies about the meaning or the consequences of his or her suicide, and can he or she distinguish fantasy from reality? What emotions are expressed about the attempt? Is he or she angry, depressed, despairing, or agitated, or is the person detached and seemingly emotionless or even pleased at the prospect of death? The less emotional the patient is, the more ominously long term the danger is.

When no attempt has yet been made, the degree of danger of the ideation must be assessed. How seriously does the patient express the wish to die as opposed to seeing it as only one way out of his or her dilemma? Is there the wish only, or has the youngster formulated a specific plan? Is the plan still only in the individual's mind, or has he or she taken steps to put it into action such as obtaining a gun or beginning to collect a perceived lethal dose of some medication? The adolescent's risk increases with each step along this continuum.

Psychiatric evaluation must be made to determine current or past existence of a mental disorder carrying increased risk of suicide. Past history of such a disorder, even if current symptoms do not exist or are equivocal, increases danger of suicide as does a history of previous suicide ideation or attempt. Is there a history of risk-taking behavior such as recklessness, antisocial activity, promiscuity, or substance use problems? A history of physical and particularly sexual abuse indicates a greater risk of suicide.

Current and recent stressors must be sought because they are often the acute precipitants of suicidality in a chronically at-risk teen. In many cases they may be less ultimately serious and therefore more immediately resolvable, thus lessening the immediate danger of an impulsive suicidal act, although the chronic risk will need continuing therapeutic attention. Have there been problems at school or in a job or in the family? Has there been trouble with the police? Has there been a recent traumatic event such as the death or loss of a parent through divorce or separation or the death or loss of a friend?

Stresses in the social context of peers are major triggers of suicidality. Adolescents who have poor relationships with their peers and thus feel isolated either chronically or through some specific recent event that has made them feel humiliated or ostracized lack the supportive structure to weather and resolve the stress. Teenagers are particularly vulnerable to sexual problems because of their great insecurity in this just-emerging and insufficiently consolidated area. Sexual difficulties can range from inability to develop and maintain a sexual relationship, or the breakup of one; inability or unwillingness to live up to the boasted sexual activity of one's peers or the perceived sexual standards of the peer group; fears of homosexual or other peer-devalued sexual impulses or fantasies; to simple confusion and helpless feelings in coping with one's own emerging sexuality. Especially for girls, but also for some of the boys involved, pregnancy or recent abortion can be an overwhelming stress. All of these aspects must be considered and when present must be included in the treatment plan.

Evaluation of the Family and Others

In assessing the family and other possible sources of support, the clinician needs to assess not only the immediate and chronic suicidal danger
for the adolescent but also the dependability of safeguards against suicide and the supports available to the youngster outside of a hospital to
make decisions about disposition. It is important to get the adolescent's
version of the family history and of what is going on within the family
involving all the various relationships as well as the family's own picture of itself. The two versions usually differ often in significant and
determinative ways. The youngster may not know the history of serious psychiatric illness in parents or close relatives that could determine
disposition when the indicators of immediate risk are equivocal, and
although the family may not appear to the evaluator to be devoid of
supportive resources, it is the youngster's perception that is real in his
or her mind and thus may determine the need for hospital protection at
least in the short term. The patient may also be more truthful than the
involved family members about physical or sexual abuse, substance
abuse, or other behaviors or conditions that would render the home environment unsafe.

Every effort should be made to get the significant family members in
for personal interviews or at the least to conduct a telephone interview
before deciding on disposition. Psychiatric and psychosocial histories are
necessary to assess genetic or historically chronic detrimental influences.
Assessment of past and present family functioning is a necessary aspect
of the total evaluation process. The unstructured family interview is most
usually done. A simple semistructured screening instrument, the family
APGAR devised by Smilkstein (1978) is a useful tool that establishes the
parameters by which a family's functional health can be measured. In the
family APGAR, five components are included: adaptation (how family
members aided each other in time of need), partnership (how family members communicate with each other about personal problems or medical
care), growth (how family members have changed during the past years),
affection (how family members have responded to emotional expressions
such as affection, love, sorrow, or anger), and resolve (how family members share time, space, and money). The instrument is designed to serve
as a guideline for management of the family in trouble.

If friends came in with a youngster, there is an opportunity to check
on how helpful and supportive or vice versa the social group can be.
Sometimes a suicidal youngster's friends are sufficiently mature and
concerned that they could remain with and monitor the patient for at

least a while even when family support is questionable or the family cannot immediately be contacted. When the family is unavailable, the clinician should proceed with the same principles of psychotherapy focusing on whatever custodial or caregiving adults are available in the adolescent's environment. At times, a friend's parents are dependable and willing to provide help and a place to stay for a limited time while ultimate disposition is being determined.

Acute Disposition

The decision to hospitalize or release a suicidal adolescent cannot be made lightly and probably should not be made alone unless the evaluator is very experienced. Judgment is especially difficult when beds are scarce, when finances or insurance force the final decision, or when family is insistent on an approach that is contrary to the evaluator's understanding.

We recommend that the evaluating psychiatrist take the most conservative and safe approach; the decision to hospitalize is always the safest. While maintaining safety, a hospital setting can offer the best opportunity to get answers to life-and-death issues about how serious the attempt was and which interventions are indicated. It can also be the initial phase of treatment. If there is any doubt or if family members could not be adequately assessed as to the safety of the environment and in the absence of alternative secure temporary arrangements, hospitalization for the protection of the patient should be mandatory. If the evaluation team believes that the circumstances do not warrant hospitalization, a follow-up visit should be scheduled usually within 24 hours. As much as possible, the evaluator should try to make a contract with the adolescent and the family regarding safety. The ongoing stage of intervention—psychotherapy or conjoint family therapy—can be decided at that time. In case of missed appointments, it is mandatory that the psychiatrist or a crisis team member—often the social worker—follow through. Continued services for actively suicidal adolescents must be offered with the same concern as the initial emergency room evaluation. Sometimes a home visit is possible and in that event, particularly enlightening.

Such determinations and measures as discussed thus far are but the first and most brief part of dealing effectively with a suicidal adolescent. Passing or even intermittent thoughts about death and suicide, unaccompanied by serious wishes, plans, or attempts are normal in older children and adolescents. However, whenever a youngster is judged to be suicidal to any serious degree, the need exists for ongoing psychiatric treatment and management. When substance abuse is a part of the overall picture, as in an adolescent who is only suicidal when under the influence of some substance or whose substance abuse is of suicidal intensity, then abuse therapy becomes a necessary, perhaps primary aspect of ongoing treatment. Acute disposition only initiates definitive mental health care. Ongoing therapy is considered in the next chapter.

6

Ongoing Treatment With
Suicidal Adolescents

This level of intervention, which we have called tertiary, occurs after the crisis of a specific suicidal act is at least temporarily past. It may take many forms and use the full existing gamut of psychotherapeutic and pharmacological modalities. Careful diagnosis of psychiatric disorders as well as understanding of the psychodynamics of suicidality are necessary to inform both the choice of therapeutic approach and the focus and conduct of therapy itself.

For example, chronic suicidal behavior is of ongoing concern to the psychotherapist and is called *characterological suicidality*. The patient uses suicidal behaviors as a way to exert omnipotent control to protect himself or herself from the sense of intense vulnerability as a result of feeling overwhelmed with hopelessness and helplessness. In contrast, the acute episodic suicidal patient has already reached or exceeded the limits of tolerance for hopelessness and helplessness, is withdrawing from others, and is acutely nonfunctional in various areas. The former requires long-term, intensive psychotherapy and firm limit setting both in everyday life and within the treatment setting (e.g., regular attendance). Interventions are aimed at explicating the omnipotence and the use of primitive, maladaptive defenses so as to channel the intense destructiveness of the patient's suicidality into the relationship with the therapist. The latter, acute style of suicidality requires a cognitive-supportive approach and often does not require long-term therapy. However, it may be that one begins to work with what appears to be an acute suicidal episode only to discover with ongoing

85

therapy that as characterological traits crystallize into character pathology, the suicidality becomes chronic.

General Principles of Therapy
Regardless of Modality

It cannot be emphasized too strongly that all modalities of therapy with adolescents, suicidal or not, are and must be based on psychodynamic understanding of the meanings of the suicidal behavior to the youngster both intrapsychically and interpersonally. Regardless of what the therapy is called—cognitive, psychoanalytic, group, or family—no therapy will bring about real change unless the therapist helps the adolescent realize what he or she was or is trying inappropriately and maladaptively to communicate or accomplish through the suicidal act. Only then can he or she reassess the goals (themselves often maladaptive) and find constructive means of achieving appropriate goals.

Diagnosis

Suicidal behaviors can be present in all types of psychiatric syndromes. The psychotherapist must have a clear diagnostic understanding of the suicidal adolescent because in most cases a suicidal patient carries a psychiatric diagnosis. If the patient is neurotic (dysthymic disorder, obsessive-compulsive disorder, hysterical), he or she has a better functioning ego than do adolescents with the more serious disorders mentioned below; an effective therapeutic alliance is more likely to be formed, and a protective nonsuicidal contract can be more trustworthy. If the patient has a personality disorder in the subgroup of impulsive personality disorders (borderline, histrionic, or antisocial), it is known that youngsters with these disorders have a high incidence of completed suicide (Stone 1990). The diagnosis of psychosis alerts one to the high incidence of suicide in schizoaffective disorder, schizophrenia, bipolar I disorder, and psychotic depression. Nonpsychotic affective disorders and panic disorder carry significant suicidal risks as do transsexualism and (especially in adolescents) homosexuality. All of these risks are intensified by substance abuse.

Appropriate biological treatments for specific psychiatric disorders, manifested by suicidal behavior, should be instituted as indicated. Discussion of these treatments is outside the focus and scope of this report.

Ongoing Assessment of Suicide Risk

Risk assessment does not relate solely to the initial interview and whatever acute intervention follows it. A systematic review of these risks should be done on an ongoing basis throughout treatment because anyone who has once been suicidal can become suicidal again. It is important, however, to underscore that it may be more difficult for the treating psychotherapist to assess suicide risk than for a consulting psychiatrist to do so. The therapist is under the influence of strong conscious and unconscious reactions to and emotions about any suicidal patient that may obscure this assessment, leading either to overestimating or underestimating suicidal risk.

The psychotherapist must assess the degree of hopelessness that the patient presents; this factor plays a most important role as predictor of risk (see Chapter 3). Hopelessness can be assessed through observation of the patient or just as importantly from the feelings of the therapist who may find himself or herself experiencing of pessimism about the treatment, the patient, and about his or her therapeutic skills (see below). This usually reflects the patient's own hopelessness about himself or herself even at times when the patient appears to be in a "good mood." This should be considered as an alerting sign by the therapist.

Sudden improvements with a sense of peace and sudden cordiality toward others (including the therapist) are a danger sign.

> Janet, a 17-year-old high school senior, had made two previous suicide attempts in the last 3 years. She was seeing a therapist once a week without clear improvement since the beginning of the academic year. She was religious and began to communicate to her therapist that she found new solace in her religion. She also decided to give away her collection of rock-and-roll cassettes, her album of photographs, and a bracelet to her closest friends. The therapist confronted her with these altruistic gestures, and the patient acknowledged she was preparing to take an overdose of pills she had accumulated. Thus the therapist and family were able to avert the suicide attempt.

Some patients make a suicide plan, which they then set aside for "emergencies." Such a plan should always be inquired about and should be dealt with in the psychotherapeutic process as a narcissistic resolution of conflicts or stresses. Such a patient has a sense of wielding omnipotent control, if not over life, then over death. Therapists must inquire in detail about patients' contingencies in the event of unfavorable circumstances.

The therapist must be alert to the anniversaries of past losses that previously destabilized a suicidal patient. Some oncoming losses as with terminally ill family members or friends can be anticipated and prepared for. Particularly with adolescents, the generally temporary nature of most of their peer relationships, especially love relationships, requires ongoing anticipatory therapeutic preparation.

Some devastating losses are internal, such as the confrontation of the loss of body function as from a disabling accident or previous suicide attempt or even impending loss of life from an incurable illness like AIDS, Huntington's chorea, or some forms of leukemia. The full awareness of aspects of the self may only come through therapy. Some psychotic patients can develop enough insight into their psychosis that a lifetime of recurrent or continuing dysfunction, misery, and hospitalization is perceived as intolerable, and this awareness may lead to suicide. Adolescents in therapy for pervasive developmental disorders may become increasingly aware of the differences between themselves and their normal peers and of the continuing negative impact their condition will have on their future lives, and they may become suicidal.

As these above circumstances are all possible as ongoing therapy progresses, the clinical assessment of suicide risk continues throughout therapy.

Interpersonal Skills

Most if not all suicidal adolescents have deficits in at least some areas of social skills. Otherwise they would have or find sufficient support from peers or adults to help them tolerate and overcome a distressing circumstance. Any therapeutic modality should include techniques or ways of approaching and addressing the bases of poor social skills and the need to build effective social interactions. Even in the psychoanalysis of adolescents, there must be enough flexibility in the analyst to direct the youngster's attention to such issues and to help him or her learn such skills.

Specific attention has been given to the relevance of peer relationships and interpersonal relationships in the discussion of suicide risk. An analysis of social skills deficits is recommended for suicidal adolescents, who generally do not know how to relate to others in age-appropriate ways. They may not be able to listen to others, or may engage others' attention only by clowning, or be unable to maintain a conversation, or not think to or know how to express appreciation or extend compliments to others when warranted.

A direct approach is helpful to assess and to clarify the person's knowledge of his or her past performance in this area of peer interaction. Performance deficits relate to problems in implementing social skills to appropriately adaptive, or acceptable, levels. Self-control skill deficits have to do with the management of emotional arousal or excitement.

Therapy should address interpersonal problem-solving skills in terms of enabling the adolescent to assess problems, to explore different scenarios of solutions and the consequences of different solutions, and to anticipate the degrees of control possible with the various scenarios. Clarification of the patient's assumptions is necessary because adolescents tend to see new things in a black-or-white fashion. An outline of this approach might be to have the patient focus on sensitivity to interpersonal problems, willingness to consider the consequences of behavior, ability to generate alternative solutions to social problems, and the ability to specify step-by-step means for attaining interpersonal goals. The support of peer groups and social interchanges with peers and friends should be stressed as peers contribute significantly to the self-esteem at this age.

Transference Issues

The unconscious perception of the therapist as being like some authority (usually parental) figure in the patient's life and the focusing of emotions and expectations on the therapist that originated in the relationship with the real parental figure are phenomena that occur with varying intensity in every therapy. This is particularly true in therapy with adolescents who under the best of circumstances are still usually deeply involved with and dependent on their parents. The blurring of boundaries between parents and therapist is intensified because it is usually a parental figure who has initiated and insisted on therapy, so that the adolescent can easily see the therapist as an extension of the parents or the parents' agent rather than his or her own agent. Whatever the parents' roles in the adolescent's final inability to cope with a life situation other than by a suicidal act, that youngster felt unable to trust them enough to turn to them for help. At some level, he or she will similarly mistrust the parent surrogate-therapist.

The suicidal adolescent will try to keep vital information secret from the therapist. He or she will expect to be understood without having to communicate clearly and in detail because parents are supposed to be omniscient. The adolescent will expect, even openly demand, immediate (magical) solutions to his or her problems and be enraged that they are not forthcoming; the therapist's "failure" to provide this may be felt as mean withholding rather than simple impossibility. Any vengeful rage toward the parents will be turned on the therapist with the inner need to hurt and defeat the source of help. The youngster may feel so help-lessly controlled by the parents or by life circumstances which he or she blames on the parents, that suicide seems like the only behavior or death the only outcome truly in his or her control, and the therapist may be-come the target of such defiant control. The adolescent may want to make the therapist feel as helpless as he or she does. The patient may be driven to punish the therapist-parent for real or imagined hurts and rejections with his or her attempted or real death.

These dynamics in various guises are ubiquitous in therapy with suicidal adolescents, although they come out in the open and lend them-selves to working through more in psychoanalytic or other therapies that focus on inner meanings rather than simply controlling or chang-ing behavior. They are no less present, however, in all therapeutic en-counters, and the therapist must be alert to them so as to bring them into the open and counteract them. The therapist is often the target for all the adolescent's transferred destructive rage and must be able to tol-erate it while helping the youngster to recognize its inappropriate focus and to moderate his or her urge toward destructive action. The thera-peutic setting must become a safe arena for the expression of the most painful and dangerous thoughts and feelings and for their exploration in thought rather than their being acted out in self-destructive behavior.

An issue related to the adolescent's perception of the therapist is that of the gender of the therapist. We are not aware of any research address-ing this issue in the context of suicidality, but it is the clinical experience of this committee that it is irrelevant in most cases. One wants the best thera-pist available regardless of gender. In instances in which the suicide at-tempt was related to sexual abuse at home or other serious conflicts with a specific parent or parent figure, it could then be important that the therapist's gender correspond with that of the safer parent. It could also be important if the adolescent specifically requested a male or female thera-pist and such a person was available and adequately qualified.

Therapists' Responses to Suicidal Adolescents

Few therapeutic challenges stir as intense and varied responses in a thera-pist as does genuine suicidality in a patient. These patients can put to test the healing capacities and positive wishes of the therapist attacking the core of the therapist's identity. By definition, a therapist is for life, not for death; is for development, not for nihilism; is for constructive, creative adaptation, not for destructive annihilation. This in turn can cause the therapist to develop an unconscious hatred toward the patient that can be expressed by unconscious malice and aversion or aloofness leading the patient to interrupt his or her treatment. The therapist's negativity, even if it reflects only pessimism rather than dislike, may be conveyed as an expectation that the patient will eventually complete a suicide attempt. Some patients may act out this perceived expectation. Any and all of the responses discussed in this section are induced by the fact of suicidality and are clearly independent of therapeutic modality. Every therapist will have human responses to such a challenge.

One hears a great deal about "countertransference" with suicidal patients as though that term subsumes all therapist responses to such patients and also as though it is somehow bad and unprofessional. Countertransference technically means a therapist's displacement onto the patient of attitudes and feelings derived from earlier situations in his or her life. As such, it is only one aspect of therapists' reaction to patients, and it can be turned to good clinical use. The vital importance of issues dealing with therapists' responses to suicidal adolescents is that they can negatively as well as positively influence therapeutic effectiveness. They demand great self-awareness and training for the therapist.

Within its accurate meaning, countertransference is a possible response to transference and is not necessarily destructive, but dangers lie in its remaining unconscious or denied. The adolescent who wants to hurt and destroy the therapist as though the therapist were the rejecting or abusive parent may elicit hurt and anger in response. The adolescent who wants to control the therapist as though the therapist were the parents by whom he or she feels controlled and helpless may produce answering helpless anxiety in the therapist. The adolescent who needs the therapist to sense his or her hopelessness and despair by making the therapist feel it himself or herself because the adolescent has never been able emotionally to elicit empathy from an insensitive parent may well set the therapist to questioning whether he or she is capable enough to do the youngster any good.

The more trained and self-aware a therapist is, the less often such responses will remain unconscious and the more fleeting the actual emotional responses will be before they trigger a new or greater understanding of the patient's psychodynamics and motives. When that happens, these reactions become powerful therapeutic tools for the therapist to use in increasing the patient's self-awareness and opening the way for the patient to explore and develop healthier options for dealing with stressful circumstances and with other people.

On the other hand, a therapist may not know why he or she is feeling angry with a patient or may try to deny that he or she could possibly have such feelings while at the same time he or she cancels appointments or fails to return phone calls. A therapist may not recognize the countertransferential basis of an anxious need to be overprotective or to hospitalize a patient unnecessarily, or of his or her buying into the youngster's need to heap all blame and responsibility on the parents as he or she tries to prove himself or herself a better and more loving parent surrogate than the patient expects him or her to be.

A therapist may become caught up in true transference conflicts of his or her own if the adolescent becomes somehow confused with a real person in their life. If the therapist is or has been a parent of adolescents, the nature and quality of the relationship with his or her children may color the responses to the patient. There may be unresolved conflicts in the therapist that are reawakened if he or she unconsciously identifies with the youngster or the parents or someone else in the drama by which that adolescent is overwhelmed to the point of suicidality.

When there is a real potential for suicide in a young patient, the specter of that disaster touches the therapist in many real and practical ways over and above any unconscious conflictual or countertransferential issues. It is so dreaded an outcome that a therapist is tempted to collude with a patient who does not want to talk about it to avoid probing for details or plans in the hope that they do not exist or will go away. Continued suicide attempts do indeed publicly demonstrate the therapist's relative ineffectiveness with that particular patient. Were actual suicide to occur, it represents therapeutic failure, and although any well-trained therapist tries to maintain a realistic sense of his or her limitations, suicide is probably the most wrenching proof of the lack of therapeutic omnipotence that one has to bear and recover from. Suicide is a complete and irrevocable rejection of all the good that the therapist has tried to offer the patient, regardless of the fact that the therapist had nothing to do with the original genesis of the suicidality.

It is not only the inner sense of value and competence that is threatened by a patient's suicidality. The therapist fears for his or her professional reputation and worries about the possibility of a lawsuit by the adolescent's parents. This latter concern is quite justified; 25% of suits against psychiatrists concern suicide and its management (F. A. Jones 1987).

Therapeutic Modalities

It is wise to make it clear in the initial consultation with a suicidal adolescent and with the family that no form of therapy, no type of medication, and no therapist has the total power to prevent suicidal behavior or completed suicide. It is fair to point out that therapy is usually successful in terms of lowering suicidality and helpful in more general terms as well and that therapy is infinitely better than no therapy. However, magical hopes as well as the tendency to place total responsibility for outcome on the therapist must be clarified from the beginning.

Types of therapy are not mutually exclusive, although they will be discussed as different entities for convenience. Because adolescence is an immature developmental stage, an adolescent even in psychoanalysis will at times require the analyst to be more of a participant in cognitive and supportive ways than may classically be expected. Furthermore, although family therapy is a specific modality when it is the principal therapeutic approach, ideally the family should be involved at some level in every therapeutic endeavor with an adolescent.

Decisions regarding implementation and timing of specific modalities of behavioral, supportive, or dynamic interventions and therapies must depend on the judgment of the therapist according to the individual needs and circumstances of each adolescent. Because there are so many individual and family variables, it is not practical to attempt a decision tree that would suggest specific therapeutic modalities to fit all specific suicidal situations. On a case-by-case basis, an assessment of which risk factors are most crucial to attend to may help to determine the most appropriate therapeutic approach at least initially. It cannot be too strongly emphasized that all intervention and treatment approaches must be sensitive to the cultural and ethnic differences that help to shape each individual patient.

Short-Term Individual Psychotherapy

Supportive and crisis intervention therapies are aimed at protecting the patient from impulsive behavior and at attenuating or eliminating factors contributing to the crisis. Patients' cognitive styles need to be addressed because a suicidal patient will show a certain inflexibility or rigidity in his or her thinking processes in regard to himself or herself, the world, and the future—all characteristically negative.

Individual psychotherapy would include a variety of approaches: cognitive, behavioral, and affective. With regard to the patient's cognitive coping style, alternative scenarios and solutions through modeling should be rehearsed in practice. This is specifically done by looking at the same problem from a different perspective, examining advantages and disadvantages, and taking different roles. In this way, cognitive alternatives that can be prepared in advance may counteract the rigid thinking that could prevail once a suicidal state recurs.

School attendance and work provide a sense of identity and accomplishment for the youngster; every effort should be made to encourage school attendance. Without a regular activity, his or her whole sense of self as a competent person whose identity is recognized by peer interaction is threatened. Encourage the youngster to volunteer for other jobs if schoolwork is not possible. A day- or after-school structured program may be indicated if the patient is not attending school.

If the patient is not psychotic or characterologically suicidal, a focus-oriented, individual, supportive type of therapy will be the treatment of choice. The patient might need to be seen on a flexible basis according to the intensity of the depression and the seriousness of the suicidal attempt, from every day to three times a week with or without family. If this cannot be accomplished, the patient may need a short period of hospitalization.

In brief problem-solving therapy for crisis intervention, the frequency of the sessions needs to be adjusted to the patient's needs. When acute suicidal danger is judged to be under control, recommendations are for outpatient treatment even with daily sessions. What is important in this respect is to provide a supportive relationship within a therapeutic alliance to concentrate on immediate specifics or concrete issues to give the patient a sense of control over his or her life. To decrease family stresses, the family has to be engaged actively as they are likely to be most receptive to the therapist's interventions at this point and may withdraw and reject efforts to work with them after the crisis is over.

An example of a short-term therapy approach that has been adapted to work with depressed adolescents is interpersonal psychotherapy (IPT). IPT is a form of individual psychotherapy that focuses on intensive work on problematic relationships through fostering an understanding of thoughts, feelings, and behaviors contributing to the conflicts in the relationships. The emphasis is on changing the patient's maladaptive interactions with significant others that are sources of stress. Although parents and other family members may be seen, the major work is done with the individual patient. The treatment follows a protocol based on a detailed treatment manual. Treatment consists of 12 weekly sessions. The key problems to be worked on are identified early in the treatment and discussion of other issues that are not considered relevant to the treatment is discouraged. In the study in which this treatment was evaluated, therapists were experienced psychiatrists or psychologists, and they underwent intensive training including supervision of videotaped sessions (Mufson et al. 1993).

Psychotherapy of any sort is not popular with adolescents or their families. A suicide attempt is shocking, it disrupts any sense of well-being in a family, and it is often thought of as a disgrace. Most youngsters and families will want to deny its importance and forget it as soon as possible. Therefore they will tend to be resistant and noncompliant with therapeutic programs after the initial interventions. Some possible strategies for such families and teenagers might be

- Brief, time-limited, focused therapy. Make an agreement for 4–6 sessions and renew if necessary, because for many families 15 sessions or more loom like an impossible task.
- Delineate to the patient what to expect, how the work will proceed, and how it could work.
- Accept and discuss it if the adolescent and his or her family want to stop earlier than agreed on. This gives them the opportunity to discuss issues before an interruption and leaves the family with a sense of control over termination that in turn may enable them to return.
- With the adolescent, prepare a list of those problems relevant to the suicidality that can be shared with important others, enlist the adolescent's cooperation in identifying those to whom it should be distributed, and urge that he or she take a role in its distribution. Such people could include the identified therapists, parents, teachers, siblings, and others. This can be an important part of the adolescent's taking responsibility and asking for help. Although this raises issues of confidentiality, in the case of an overt suicide attempt, the attempt is usually already to some degree public knowledge and in general the safety of the child is primary, confidentiality secondary. This is one standard behavioral technique that is frequently used by members of this committee. This list could also serve to prioritize what problems must be addressed first.
- Prepare a written statement of goals and new skills for problem solving for circulation to the same people.

Long-Term Psychoanalytic Therapy

Psychoanalysis and intensive psychoanalytic therapy are treatment modalities significantly different from the brief, crisis-focused, cognitive- and behavior-oriented therapies. The difference lies not in its focus on psychodynamics, because all competent therapy of suicidal adolescents must take into account the meanings of the suicidal behavior to the specific, individual patient. The difference lies mostly in the depth to which these dynamics are explored and reawakened in the intense and long-lasting therapeutic encounter and in the noninterventional stance of the analyst.

Psychoanalysis is currently probably the least used therapeutic modality for adolescent suicidality. Not many adolescents are appropriate subjects for analysis. There is an increasing social pressure for more rapid results; other modalities would usually have to be employed first to take care of the emergency nature of much of adolescent suicidality; and the insurance climate is hostile to long-term, in-depth therapy. However, analytic concepts form one of the important bases of long-term inpatient treatment. In addition, there are some issues of personality structure and conflict resolution that often remain unaddressed in less deep-going therapy.

In analysis, the conflict-, trauma-, and deficit-based unconscious distortions, fantasies, fears, and wishes are reelicited in their original intensity and come to focus on the analyst and to be acted out or reexperienced in the therapeutic relationship. This means there is greater regression in such therapy, with much transient dependency, and the risk of increased depression and suicidality. For this reason, only those adolescents judged to have adequate ego strength and family and social resources may be appropriate for analytic therapy. It is in this reexperiencing of the original causes and sources of psychopathology in a benign and caring relationship that the adolescent can work through and resolve them and emerge with healthier ego development than was possible in his or her original family milieu. The periods of intensification of the suicidality can seriously test the analyst's judgment regarding the youngster's basic ego strength and may at times require hospitalization to ensure the patient's safety.

In classic analysis, the analyst takes no role in the patient's life outside of the therapeutic interaction in the office. No suggestions about real life are made, and hospitalizations, even medication, are turned over to a colleague. Some adolescents can tolerate and benefit from such austerity.

However, there is growing awareness in the analytic community that adolescents are still children in many ways. They are not yet past real developmental needs for supportive, guiding adult (parental) relationships. They may not be able to obtain appropriate satisfaction of these real—not neurotic—needs in the family milieu in which the problems originally developed or from other adults in their lives. There is increasing sensitivity in the analytic field to the need for the analyst to be a real person for an adolescent. In many instances, even when the adolescent has the ego capacity for working through pathology at the deepest of levels, classic analysis is too interpersonally distant an interaction. Such interpersonal reserve constitutes real, not just transferential, indifference and rejection. The analyst may often need to be able to move back and forth between more and less interactive positions to help the adolescent achieve optimum therapeutic results.

DSM-III (American Psychiatric Association 1980), DSM-III-R (American Psychiatric Association 1987), and DSM-IV (American Psychiatric Association 1994) may have done psychotherapy a grave disservice by eliminating the concept of neurosis. Although neurosis may be difficult to define with research rigor, it is seen daily by dynamically aware psychiatrists. *Neurosis* refers to psychiatric conditions in patients with deep-seated conflicts or deficit-based disorders that are not of severe character pathology degree; such patients constitute the main group for whom analysis is often the treatment of choice. If psychiatrists limit their conceptual breadth to the diagnostic categories recognized since DSM-III, it could appear that character pathology constitutes the only group of patients for whom analysis may be appropriate or necessary. Although analysis is indeed a valid therapeutic modality for such teenagers, their prognosis is often poor compared with that of neurotic adolescents.

The following condensed summary of the 3.5-year analysis of a girl who began therapy at age $15^1/_2$ is one example of analytic therapy. She was seen five times a week using the technique of lying on the couch (P. Kernberg 1974).

> Alicia was the first child of an excessively close Spanish immigrant family. Her father was a professional extremely involved in his profession and emotionally distant at home. Her mother was a constricted person, severely obese, experiencing conversion symptoms, and overinvolved and overidentified with her children. Alicia had a minor facial scar from difficult forceps delivery, but her early childhood was normally uneventful until the first of her siblings was born when she was 2 years old. Her relations with her parents became increasingly strained, and she began to

have intense, long lasting temper tantrums that continued up to the time of psychiatric referral.

She had been a good student but a loner in school. Menarche occurred at age 13, and she was both afraid of and embarrassed by her periods. She was disgusted by the idea of sexual intercourse and stated she would never marry or have children. She had asthma and numerous allergies, which she used both to gain her father's attention and to rationalize her avoidance of dating. Suicidal threats at home, during which several times she put a jump rope around her neck, prompted her referral to a psychiatrist. Alicia was in full agreement; she wanted help.

At the time of her evaluation, her low self-esteem was graphically portrayed by her moderate obesity, general unkempt appearance, and a general demeanor of not deserving the space she occupied. However, there was much that indicated good ego strength. Her superior intelligence, verbal ability, potential access to her emotions, awareness of discomfort and desire for help, sense of humor, and ability to use her capacities in other activities such as art indicated she had the ego capacities to participate in psychoanalysis, which was considered the treatment of choice.

The theme of death was brought up within the first few sessions and remained a constant theme until termination. Death and suicide had multiple layers of meanings for Alicia, and the different meanings arose and shifted back and forth throughout. Initially it reflected her devalued sense of self and the conviction that no one cared for her, and everyone—parents, friends, school, analyst—would be better off without her. As angry feelings toward her parents began to emerge, suicide meant expiation for unacceptable rage as well as a way to hurt them. There were several mild to moderate suicide gestures (wrist scratching and cutting) during this early period—a communication through behavior rather than words. Her wishes to become someone valuable and useful in life were contaminated by the fantasy of omnipotent power to hurt others, and she came to fear violent retaliation; suicide meant she, not feared others, was in control of life or death.

She began to deal with her hatred of her body, her menses, her femaleness. There was clear evidence of unconscious fantasies that she had been castrated. She feared her sexuality, was guilty about sex play with siblings, and was ashamed of her fascination with her father's nudity. She equated that with incest and equated all boys with her father so she dared not date. Suicide also meant expiation for bad sexual feelings.

By the second year of analysis, she was dealing intensively with her angers and hostile aggression and her fears of destroying others through her omnipotent powers. This was now transferred fully on the analyst, and her rage was projected on the analyst as someone who wanted to ruin and spoil everything for her. Much of her rage derived from the analyst's failure to fulfill her desire for total infantile gratification, and this caused guilt over her voracious demandingness. There was a crisis of suicidality and suicidal gestures resulting from an occasion when Alicia expressed anger by wanting to terminate, and immediately thereafter the analyst became ill. Suicide would punish them both, she for her devouring anger, and the analyst for her withholding gratification.

Guilty conflict over female sexuality intensified as she revealed that she had been masturbating, a great sin in her eyes, since before analysis began. She used a flashlight given to her by her father and used it vigorously enough to produce both erotic pleasure and some bleeding. Masturbatory guilt turned out to be a deeper motive for her earlier suicidality, which had precipitated her referral for therapy. Death would also protect the good aspects of her parents and analyst from her dangerous badness.

By the third year, the chronic escalation of her verbal attacks on the analyst reached the point at which protective hospitalization was considered, although it never became necessary. There was great rage at having to accept that neither the analyst (parents) nor herself was omnipotent enough to protect her from all future uncertainties. She could tolerate such rage only by thinking of killing herself as punishment at the same time.

The working through of these conflicts was also beginning to produce positive results. She was beginning to accept herself as a female. She began to see beyond her suicidality to a positive and good future that would be destroyed by death. Furthermore, as her analyst began to emerge as a real person for whom she could feel interest and concern—not only a transference object—her suicide threats ceased.

There was a temporary surge of suicidal threats and wishes when Alicia discovered that her analyst was pregnant. This brought out her hateful envy of her parents' intimacy from which she was excluded, and suicide represented a sadistic attack on her mother for being her father's sex partner and for producing the siblings who destroyed her sole claim on her parents' affection.

Alicia terminated after the analyst had given birth. She had by then lost weight and was dressing well and looking attractive, and she had begun to date. She was quite articulate in dealing with the sadness and loss of terminating and about the real and beneficial changes that analysis had brought about.

Group Therapy

Group therapy at a time when a youngster is at acute risk of suicidal behavior is contraindicated because most adolescent groups do not have the flexibility to accommodate to the patient's precarious equilibrium with the concern and availability of attention that the patient requires. After the acute crisis has been resolved, group therapy can be helpful in supportive ways in terms of developing social and problem-solving skills. Individual therapy and group therapy can complement each other; they are not mutually exclusive.

Group therapy for adolescents not in crisis has long been recognized as having valuable application at this life stage. Adolescents are more comfortable in a group of age peers; they feel less at a child-parent disadvantage than they do one-to-one with an adult therapist. It is possible to move in and out of verbal participation (according to individual readiness) when there are others to talk. Other adolescents are particularly sharp at picking up each other's tricks, games, and evasions, and a youngster can hear a confrontation by a peer with much less defensiveness than from a parent-like adult. Once some inappropriate or maladaptive response is in the open, the therapist can pick up on it and foster its exploration. Group therapy is also uniquely valuable in helping the participants develop the social skills that are so frequently lacking in suicidal adolescents.

Forbes (1972) describes how, in a group session with suicidal adolescents who had been involved in incestuous relationships, they progressively became aware of the hatred and anger expressed in the suicidal act—first by seeing it in the other members, then in themselves.

Kay: "I want to tell you all something I've never said before. Why did my father kill himself when I did try to satisfy him (sexually)? I didn't give enough. He killed himself because of me!" she cried. Her entire body quivered. The room was hushed.

Therapist: "Kay, your father didn't kill himself because of your not satisfying him. I think you can see, though, how angry one is when one takes his life. You felt that if he really loved you he would not have done it. He would not have done it if he had not been thinking so much of himself. But he did, and you feel *that* to be his anger and rejection of you. I can imagine he must have felt very guilty over his seduction of you." Kay broke down hysterically. She was given a drink of water and a mild tranquilizer.

At once, in different ways, those who had attempted suicide asked, "Did my folks feel that way when I tried to kill myself? Did my parents think I blamed them? Is that why my parents were so upset?"

Carol: "I never realized before that my mother could think I was mad at her. All I felt was that I wanted to get away. How terrible."

Bea: "I knew I felt mad, but I just didn't want to live. I felt I couldn't do anything right. I'm just not important to anyone."

Therapist: "Bea, you're demonstrating how angry you were at yourself because you couldn't feel anger toward them. As you say, you were unimportant. It's yourself you feel hatred for, but you've been angry at them. You have often told me how guilty you are that you cannot do anything to please your father, yet you are angry at his demands."

Kay: "But how can you know he didn't do it because I couldn't satisfy him? He kept telling me he'd kill himself if I didn't."

Carol: "I took the pills to get away, but I know I've wished my sister was dead. I was angry at my mother for favoring her."

Therapist: "Kay, your father may have been very angry at your mother, or felt rejected by her, in that he became involved with you. Remember how unimportant you felt, and his attention to you made you feel better."

Carol: "But Kay, you have to understand that when we tried to commit suicide, we didn't feel we wanted to hurt anyone."

Kay: "But I feel I'm to blame."

Bea: "Kay, when you feel unimportant and bad you don't think of anyone else."

Therapist: "I think this is all very important. Those of you who have attempted suicide see how the others feel. Kay, you also can be aware that the person who attempts it does not necessarily think at the moment of hurting someone, though that's what happens. It is a very angry act, though it does not seem that way."

Lou: "My father is still alive, and I can't get along with my mother. She is always sitting on his lap in front of me. I get very upset. Is it because of what happened?"

Therapist: "You feel angry that she reminds you that she is his wife. You also feel guilty about ever having become involved with him. When you steal and get in trouble—and you notice you make sure you are caught—you are punishing yourself and them at the same time, much as Kay's father did."[1]

Sugar (1972) described what he called network therapy, in which the therapist explicitly invites the adolescent patient to bring age-peer friends to his or her sessions so as to enhance his or her relationships with other people and to counteract the risk of suicide or hospitalization. Once the adolescent is deemed able to deal with the suicidal crisis by his or her capacity to exert genuine self-control and by his or her honest interaction with the therapist, the adolescent is asked whether

---

[1]Reprinted from Forbes LM: "Incest, Anger, and Suicide," in *Adolescents Grow in Groups.* Edited by Berkovitz IH. New York, Brunner/Mazel, 1972. Used with permission.

he or she would like to have a group or therapeutic club of his or her own, having friends—as many and as often as he or she wants—and choosing them himself or herself. The family's permission is requested with the explanation that friends can provide helpful information or experiences. The fee per session remains the same, the friends are not charged, confidentiality is kept by the therapist, and their contacts outside the sessions remain as before. The peer group sessions range from 1 to 10, and the friends' attendance may fluctuate.

Generally, the patient chooses one or more healthier, more mature friends. Not surprisingly in the group sessions, arising from genuine concern, friends can express anger or disgust about the suicidal behavior, which is a powerful confrontation mediated by the therapist. At times this therapeutic strategy may serve as a turning point to the patient who uses the peer as a healthier aspect of himself or herself as an ego ideal.

The principle of patient-selected group membership provides a source of control for the patient and enhanced self-esteem. The choice of a peer or peers in turn reflects the current stage of therapy in that a problematic peer will reflect the patient's resistances. In contrast, a healthier peer may reflect the patient's own aspirations for improvement.

In sum, peer group therapy has been used for suicidal adolescents as an adjunct to other modalities. It is usually brief, 1 to 10 sessions, and it has a positive effect on locus of control, self-esteem, and autonomy even in those instances when a peer who has a negative influence on the patient is invited. In such an instance, the potential for extricating oneself from an enmeshed peer relationship is enhanced by the presence of an objective third person, the therapist. A flexible approach to the use of individual, family, or peer group therapy may be indicated and can be useful when the therapist considers using important figures in the patient's life as possible participants in family or self-selected peer group sessions.

Family Therapy

Whenever possible, the family should be involved in therapeutic work with a suicidal adolescent. In other modalities of therapy, the adolescent is considered the patient, and work with the family is adjunctive. In family therapy as a specific modality, the family is considered the patient and the adolescent is the (current) symptom bearer. Family therapy in this sense derives from the systems perspective on health and dysfunction. There are a number of approaches to family therapy; what follows is meant to present general principles.

The family systems perspective on healthy or dysfunctional adolescent development was discussed in Chapter 2. The systems perspective with regard to therapy views causality as circular, complex, and the product of multiple influences and interdependent processes. The influence of life events is mediated by multiple variables—meanings, relationships, contexts—most importantly the family's organizational patterns, meaning systems, and coping responses (Bateson 1972; Hoffman 1981). Symptoms in the individual family member are regarded as an expression of family dysfunction, an inability to respond adaptively to external stress and developmental challenge while providing protection and nurturance to family members.

The following vignette demonstrates the enmeshment of an adolescent's suicidal ideation and behavior in overall family pathology.

Marsha, a 16-year-old, was referred for therapy by her pediatrician for family difficulties and a recent drop in grades. During the first interview, she described existential concerns, had increasingly become more rebellious at school, and seemed unduly attached to her mother. She increasingly resented her authoritarian, explosive, short-tempered father, had dyed her hair, was dressing provocatively, and was causing concern in her school because of her "heavy" makeup. Her mother secretly supported her behavior. The father seemed both enraged and fascinated by his daughter's recent behavior.

During the first few interviews, Marsha confessed to occasional suicidal ideation framed in an existential, anhedonic, and intellectualized manner. She denied any other difficulties except her resentment and anger at her father. On closer inspection, she confessed to having had a few mild car accidents; she liked to drive fast. She denied any drug or substance abuse. Even though she dressed provocatively, she was afraid of men and had never had a boyfriend.

The family was initially hesitant to be involved in family therapy so an evaluation of the individual family members was done. The father confessed he had had many relationships during his lifetime, all of them younger women. He was authoritarian and was the sole economic provider at home. The mother had become increasingly depressed and detached, finding solace in reading morbid poems and sharing her readings with her daughter for the last couple of years. She had few other interests, was overeating, and had sleeping difficulties. She felt trapped and unable to leave the marriage because of the children and felt she was getting to the "end of the rope." She suspected that her husband had many sexual liaisons but was not sure about this and had discussed it with Marsha. She denied any suicidal attempts.

During the process of evaluation, Marsha got into a serious accident, luckily without any physical harm. During the session after the accident, Marsha was actively suicidal. The therapist had recommended that the parents come as well and left sufficient time for an immediate reassessment. An individual session was immediately implemented with the mother who confessed she had been having recurrent dreams that she and her daughter had had a car accident, died, and gone to heaven. She was then free of pain and her husband "had been duly punished." When the therapist saw the father, he seemed very upset and informed the therapist that in attempting to break up with his recent lover the day before his daughter's accident, his lover had made a suicide attempt by an overdose. This and his daughter's recent accident was too much to bear. However, he showed no insight into the sequence of events and denied any problems of his own except an explosive temper.

Hospitalization for the daughter was recommended with a strong recommendation of a family therapy approach. On follow-up, the daughter remained in the hospital for a short stay and continued individual therapy; the parents entered couple treatment. On a 6-month follow-up the parents had decided to separate. The mother had started to work, and Marsha was doing well in school and engaged in many peer-related extracurricular activities. The father continued to be involved with his children and was reassessing his relationships with women.

In this case, there was no history of impulsivity, substance abuse, overt depression, overt losses, and no previous history of overt suicide attempts in the adolescent. "Driving fast," "an existential emptiness," sudden changes in academic performance, and occasional suicidal thoughts were some of the early signals. The real understanding of the case, nevertheless, would not have been possible if the family had not been carefully evaluated. The mother's own suicidal ideation, chronic depressive feelings, and overinvolvement with her daughter and the father's ambivalent feelings toward his daughter and wife constituted in this case the "real" risk factors and were crucial in implementing an appropriate treatment approach and eventual symptom resolution. Just as suicidality is symptomatic of a variety of individual diagnoses and an expression of the failure of coping strategies and adaptive mechanisms, so suicidality in an adolescent family member may be a final common pathway reflecting a variety of patterns of family interaction. The completed suicide or the suicidal act or gesture may be construed as an act of aggression, manipulation, defiance, suffering and pain, a cry for help, an attempt at reconciliation and reunion, or a desperate move toward separation. Whatever the multidimensional meanings of the act, the family context and perspective greatly enrich one's understanding of them. Landau-Stanton and Stanton (1985) have suggested that it is important to view suicide as a possibly sacrificial and certainly a transactional occurrence rooted in family dynamics. Meanings will be constructed out of the conversations and narratives among family members and clinicians where the meanings attributed to the event are seen as a reflection of family structure, belief system, affect, and pattern of communication. Reflection on these variables and interventions guided by the cooperative reflection constitute the family therapy approach.

The Crisis and the Question of Hospitalization

Assessment of the suicidal adolescent brings the clinician, in consultation with the family, to a decision concerning the level of risk and the need for hospitalization. This has been addressed from other perspectives elsewhere in this report. As exemplified in the vignette above, the decision to admit the index patient needs to follow an assessment of the family with particular attention to the following.

- *Structure and stability:* What is the family's capacity to supervise and protect the adolescent? Is there a stable parental coalition, a family support system, resources to organize around the family function of protection of the young? Does the family need a respite?
- *Family affect:* Are one or both parents angry at the suicidal adolescent, overwhelmed, distraught, panic-stricken, and unable to manage their own feelings?
- *Communication:* Are the adolescent and family able to communicate openly, address the issue of safety, and enter into a safety contract? However the question of hospitalization is answered, the decision-making process must include the family, for the response to the stress event is revealing of the family dynamics and the involvement of the family is the beginning of engaging the family in treatment.

Systemic Engagement

In addition to the engagement of the suicidal adolescent and family in the treatment process, work with adolescents with a high degree of risk and severity of psychopathology requires the collaboration of an extensive system of professionals and helpers that frequently will have gathered around the adolescent. The network will frequently include outpatient therapists, teachers and school counselors, agencies, clergy, and probation officers. To avoid undermining treatment, it is essential that all clinicians and helpers agree on common goals. This is achieved during the initial phase of treatment by including the adolescent's network in an early family meeting, particularly during a time-limited course of treatment.

The Safety Contract and the Safety Watch

As the suicidal act constitutes a family crisis and a psychiatric emergency, emergency intervention is required. As described above, assessment of the adolescent and family will lead to a decision concerning hospitalization. In cases where a collaborative decision is made not to hospitalize, a written safety contract is developed by the family, the suicidal adolescent, and the clinician. A safety contract may include the around-the-clock supervision of the adolescent by the family with the support and involvement of extended family and friends. A safety contract begins with a verbalized commitment from the adolescent patient to cooperate and communicate. Cooperation in this context means a commitment to let a family member know if the intensity of suicidal impulses escalates. The family's commitment is to provide supervision at all times and to consult with their therapists at any time. The commitment of the therapists is to help the family determine its resources and support systems, organize itself and its support system, and design a detailed plan for the safety watch. The cardinal rule is that the patient will be within view of a member of the watch at all times.

Landau-Stanton and Stanton (1985) have developed the family safety watch as a family intervention with self-destructive adolescents for both outpatient and inpatient settings. In the inpatient setting, the family replaces staff in providing the around-the-clock safety checks, creating a schedule in collaboration with the unit staff. The primary aim of this method, according to the authors, is to mobilize the family to competently take care of its own.

Modifying or terminating the family watch is decided by family, adolescent, and therapists with the inpatient treatment team. This decision is made using behavioral criteria that reflect diminished suicidality and increased use of adaptive mechanisms for affect regulation, including taking personal responsibility, demonstrating more open communication, age-appropriate behavior, and improved relationships with parents and siblings.

The safety watch, a first step in the family therapy of the suicidal adolescent, serves several important functions:

- It empowers a family that may feel helpless and offers the family a vehicle for recreating hopefulness where there had been doubt and hopelessness.
- It strengthens the parental coalition and reestablishes generational boundaries while reconnecting the nuclear family and the extended family. Thus, it begins the process of differentiation of the enmeshed family and engagement of a disengaged family.
- It offers a context in which denied themes and affects may be articulated, surfaced, and addressed openly.

An intervention as intensive as the safety watch may convey the expectation that the adolescent will be unable to control his or her suicidality and thus backfire by inducing the patient to act out that expectation. Although there is always uncertainty, this countertherapeutic consequence has not been seen by those who use this technique.

Initial and Early Interventions

The first sessions of family therapy after hospitalization decisions and plans for the safety of the adolescent address the family history with a focus on the following.

Transitional mapping. Landau (1982) defined this as assessing the family's place along the transitional points of the life cycle, including changes in home and neighborhood, economic status, family composition as with the emancipation of an older sibling, and relationships with extended family, particularly the grandparental generation.

Of all nodal transitions, losses within the family of suicidal adolescents, both recent and remote, are particularly significant and constitute a major risk factor. Recent and unresolved death of a grandparent may not only bring grief to the adolescent but also a pervasive depression to the parent and the family system. Not infrequently, the death of a grandparent brings to the surface unresolved affects in the bereaved parent leading to a long period of emotional unavailability of that parent for the children, producing a second, more subtle loss.

Remote losses of significance with suicidal adolescents such as the death of a sibling, particularly an older sibling with whom the adolescent has been closely identified, seem to contribute to vulnerability. Not uncommonly, the index patient is seen by the family as a successor to a deceased family member and is invested with the characteristics of that relative. This is particularly true in families where the deceased significant family member was a completed suicide.

Cross-sectional focus.   In addition to the longitudinal transitional mapping, information is obtained concerning current family life-cycle events, conflicts, and changes. Current stressors will exacerbate long-standing vulnerabilities. These events obtain their meaning within the context of the family's life-cycle trajectory and from the various relationships of the suicidal act of the adolescent, the current family stressors, and nodal life-cycle events. These meanings and relationships will be the basis on which family therapy will proceed.

Various Approaches to Further Family Therapy

In the structural-strategic approach to the family therapy as described by Landau-Stanton and Stanton (1985), various forms of reframing or "positive interpretation" are used to diffuse the paralyzing affects and rigidity of suicidal families in crisis. Thus, the family therapist will praise the noble intentions or sacrificial aspect of the self-destructive behaviors of the adolescent, pointing out how this desperate act brought the family the attention it needed. This reframing may be particularly important where the suicidal behavior is linked to unresolved grief over losses in the family (Paul and Grosser 1965). Here the suicidal adolescent may be viewed as the repository of family grief, the mourner and martyr. Constructing this metaphor and thereby making the affects more explicitly articulated allows the family to engage in the necessary family grieving.

Psychoanalytically oriented approaches to family therapy focus on the meanings of suicidal behavior with an emphasis on dynamic issues and shared unconscious fantasies and affects. From this family dynamic perspective, adolescent suicide is a response to specific unconscious dynamic issues within the family. A shared family regression during the adolescence of a particular child may evoke in the child unconscious connections between the early care of his or her body and current needs for parental protection. Parental regression and lack of responsiveness in interaction with the child's fantasies and ego deficits may evoke an unbearable rage or feelings of abandonment that may eventuate in self-destruction (Shapiro and Freedman 1987).

Whatever the approach, as the family therapy of the suicidal adolescent proceeds, there remain essential issues to be explored and articulated, including

- Structural issues including the boundary phenomena such as enmeshment or disengagement the strength of the parental coalition and the intergenerational boundaries as well as family rituals, routines, rules, discipline, and limit setting;
- Communication and affect regulation issues including empathy, warmth, receptivity, and the articulation of loving or angry affects without projection, blaming, or the failure to take personal responsibility; and
- Conflict resolution and problem-solving issues, including the family's capacity to resolve conflict and solve problems while taking into account individual family members' needs, differences, and limitations, as well as time and context.

The foregoing discussion and general principles involve intricate and complex considerations and are most applicable to family therapy approaches that are likely to be lengthy and open ended. To deal with suicidal adolescents and their families in circumstances in which long-term therapy is impossible or impractical, S. Miller et al. (1992) have developed a structured, six-session technique for suicide attempters that incorporates family systems orientation into cognitive-behavioral approach. Their comprehensive manual provides detailed instructions for the sessions.

The basic assumption is that a suicide attempt is a response to unsolved family problems resulting from stress or intergenerational conflicts. In such dysfunctional families, crises (including suicide attempts) are seen as emergencies that protect the families from the pain of confronting difficult, basic dilemmas. Such resistance to change is seen as a commitment to support the family. Each of the six sessions has distinct and different goals and specific techniques for accomplishing them. The therapy focuses on identifying strengths in the family, on solving the interpersonal conflicts, on lowering the likelihood of maladaptive maneuvers such as suicide attempts, and on planning for coping with future suicidal crises.

Long-Term Residential Treatment

The borderline suicidal adolescent (Stone 1990), whose pathology is linked with incest four times more often than that of bipolar and schizophrenic adolescents, must be removed from his or her family for obvious reasons. Furthermore, in cases where incest is not the cause of borderline suicidality, the severity of the psychopathology and risk and the intensity of and problems inherent in the therapy of such a condition argue in favor of removal to a more controlled full-time environment. The goal is to rehabilitate the youngster in his or her social interactions by providing new opportunities to form healthier patterns of friendship, to prevent repetitive patterns of acting out sexual behavior, and to counteract self-defeating and self-destructive acts, of which suicide is the extreme. In general, long-term and intensive psychotherapy of severe character pathology goes best in the context of long-term relationships with the same therapists and therapeutic team.

Most importantly, the staff should be constantly prepared to accept the high risk involved in this solution and to alert each other (and responsible family or guardians) that suicide is an ongoing risk. The adolescent may then have the possibility of internalizing this concern and making himself or herself responsible, thus negating the fantasy of omnipotent control by the staff. In turn the staff is protected from playing into omnipotent rescue fantasies that sooner or later contribute to staff burnout and from developing counteraggression expressed through overt or covert rejection of the patient.

Long-term supportive-expressive psychotherapy should be recommended when available as an ongoing measure to neutralize the long-term effects of trauma in the life of these patients.

Partial hospitalization refers to a type of treatment that involves intensive programming similar to that found in inpatient settings, but only during a part of the day and usually 5 days per week. Patients continue to live at home while they attend the program. Programs serving adolescents usually include an on-site school and provide group and family therapy as the major treatment modalities. Partial hospitalization is generally used to provide a transition from inpatient to outpatient treatment for patients who have been hospitalized or as an alternative to hospital treatment for those for whom outpatient treatment has been insufficient. Partial hospitalization is appropriate for the suicidal adolescent who is able to contract for safety. Families must be able to support the adolescent's involvement in the treatment. Close monitoring of the suicidal symptoms, with frequent psychiatric assessment, is important. The immediate availability of a hospital is crucial because such patients may decompensate and need emergency hospitalization.

Postvention

Postvention refers to "working with survivor victims of a completed suicide to help them with their anguish, guilt, anger, shame, and perplexity" (H. N. Brown 1989). Interventions at this level, after a completed suicide has occurred, mean therapeutic work with surviving family members, friends, possibly other important and emotionally involved people such as teachers, and—not at all least—with the adolescent's therapist and therapeutic team.

Families that are not so psychologically distant as to refuse postventive involvement can be worked with regarding feelings such as guilt and remorse, aloofness, and the sense of stigmatization. Resnick (1969) has described work with such a family as fostering a process of psychological resynthesis, composed of resuscitation (dealing with the immediate wound to the survivors), rehabilitation (working through the mourning process), and renewal (giving up bondage to the suicide). A major reason for urging families to participate in postsuicide therapy and a major goal of postvention is to try to anticipate and prevent the development of posttraumatic stress disorder in family members.

Therapeutic work, often in the school setting with peer groups and friends of the youngster, deals also with many of the same guilt-ridden reactions that family members have. It may prevent a cluster of suicides or suicide attempts. Therapeutic work also can provide an opportunity to counteract the effects of the media on the youngsters in terms of idealizing or even glorifying the deceased. Depending on the circumstances of the suicide or the teacher-student milieu in the school, teachers and other adults may be included in student groups or worked with separately. Unless any particular survivors develop a specific psychiatric condition in consequence of the suicide, postventive work is usually done with groups of survivors rather than with individuals (though parents and siblings may initially benefit from individual attention). Many communities also have more or less organized self-help survivor groups, and although there are potential risks from groups that deal with potentially dangerous emotions but are not carefully and competently professionally supervised, in general such groups are usually quite valuable to the participants.

This report has already discussed the reactions of therapists to suicidal adolescents. With a completed suicide, the response of the therapist is infinitely more intense and debilitating. There are few relevant studies and perhaps none specifically addressing the therapist and adolescent suicide. The studies available (H. N. Brown 1987a, 1987b, 1989; F. A. Jones 1987; Litman 1965; Maltsberger 1992) reported both emotional and practical consequences. In addition to the pain, anger, rejection, and loss of self-esteem, the therapist's emotions, and those of colleagues, may leave him or her feeling isolated just when he or she most needs support. Some therapists require years to overcome the experience plus additional personal therapy to rebuild a sense of professional competence. Some decide never again to work with suicidal or severely depressed patients. Even in the absence of specific practice limitations, the experience will color future interactions with patients, often in unconsciously negative ways.

Training programs have the structure in which it is potentially easier to provide the necessary interventions for trainees and supervisors (see Chapter 7), although they rarely do so in any adequate fashion. Such postventions are just as vital for therapists out in practice, but a preexisting structure for it rarely exists except possibly for hospital-based therapists. Every effort should be made by local professional societies or by the therapist himself or herself if necessary to recognize the importance of developing some form of peer interaction at least to help the therapist survivor deal with the immediate and ongoing impact of a patient suicide.

7

Training Issues

The goals of early identification of adolescents at risk, management of suicidal behaviors, appropriate treatment for related emotional or psychiatric disorders, and prevention of suicide can only be attained through the final common pathway of caregivers who are adequately trained in the diverse issues that have been discussed in the previous chapters.

The concepts of primary, secondary, and tertiary prevention provide a useful framework for examining training needs for a broad, comprehensive model of prevention, management, and treatment of suicidal behaviors in youth. If the suicide of a young person is to be prevented, that person must be identified as potentially suicidal, the identified youth must be offered and accept a treatment, and the treatment must be successful.

The early identification of adolescents at risk for suicidal behaviors requires training of individuals most likely to come into contact with at-risk youth. These so-called gatekeepers come into contact with youngsters on a regular basis, have the opportunity to observe their behavior over time, and may facilitate adolescents' entry into the health care system. The Report of the Secretary's Task Force on Youth Suicide (U.S. Department of Health and Human Services 1989b) identifies a number of gatekeepers, including parents, school personnel, friends, youth group leaders, clergymen, and primary care physicians. Other important gatekeepers include social service and juvenile justice system staff. The educational needs of parents, friends, school staff, and community in general can be understood in the context of community primary prevention, which is discussed in Chapter 5.

Health professionals are often in positions where they may serve both as gatekeepers and as providers of continuing care for high-risk and suicidal youth. This chapter addresses the issue of training needs in the general health and mental health disciplines of caregivers to adolescents and their families at several points along the continuum of risk for suicidal behaviors.

Background

Adolescents are the only segment of the United States population in which mortality rates have not declined rapidly during the past decades (Fingerhut and Kleinman 1989). Most (73%) of the mortality in this group has been attributed to intentional and unintentional injuries and violence. The general health care system has been identified as an important part of a community system to address the prevention and management of problems related to injury mortality, including suicide (Perrin et al. 1992). Unfortunately, there are many barriers to effective use of traditional health services by adolescents, including discomfort with traditional settings that may not accommodate developmental needs for autonomy and privacy, lack of insurance or money to cover costs of care, and travel and scheduling barriers. In addition, among the adolescents at highest risk for poor health outcomes, including suicide, are homeless and runaway youths who face even more formidable obstacles to access to services.

Despite the difficulties in access, physicians, nurses, and other health care professionals in settings such as emergency departments and general medical and prenatal clinics do come in contact frequently with at-risk youth. Disturbed youths in particular may not seek help in the medical setting. Furthermore, the physical needs of young people are generally the focus of attention in these settings; it is known that psychological, school, or family problems often go unrecognized by many health care providers (Costello 1988). Cohen et al. (1991) found that adolescents rarely discussed their behavioral and emotional problems with physicians and that physicians did not often refer adolescents to mental health specialists. In a study of 2,787 inner-city adolescents, where reports of mental and physical health problems as well as use of clinic services were examined, analysis of selected patient problems revealed that only one-half of subjects with major depression sought or received care for depression. Less than one-third of those with suicidal ideation, conduct disorder, or substance abuse sought or received care for these problems (Stiffman et al. 1988). A British study of 50 adolescent suicide attempters found that 50% had visited their physician during the month prior to their attempt and 25% had visited 1 week prior to their attempt (Hawton et al. 1982). They had been admitted to general hospitals during the previous year at a rate three times that expected for the general British pediatric population. Although 30% of the attempters in this group had had a previous episode of self-injury, only one-third of them had been referred for treatment. Although 20% had received prescriptions for psychotropic medication during their visits, only 10% reported having discussed the problems related to their suicide attempt. This study suggests both the tremendous potential and the current difficulties in identification of suicidal youth within general health care settings.

Another factor that adds importance to the role of the general health care setting in the identification and provision of services to youngsters at risk for suicide is the possible relationship between chronic illness and suicidal behaviors. Children with epilepsy appear to be at higher risk, although the issue is not settled (Brent 1986; Kim 1991). Some uncontrolled studies of suicide completers (Sathyavathi 1975) and of attempters (Hawton et al. 1982) have found a rate of physical illness higher than that expected for the general population of adolescents. Other studies of suicide completers have not described an increased rate (Chia 1979; Shaffer 1974). As AIDS becomes more prevalent in the adolescent population, this disorder may also contribute to the suicide risk in adolescence as it does in older groups (Marzuk et al. 1988).

Epidemiological studies of adolescent community samples also suggest that although many youngsters at risk are seen in the health care system, only a modest proportion actually seek help for their emotional or behavioral problems within the general health care system (Offord et al. 1987; K. Smith and Crawford 1986; Whitaker et al. 1990). In any case, the general health care setting remains an important setting for identification of at-risk youth, although probably to a lesser extent than for adults because of the relatively greater importance of the school and other community settings for identification of risk and provision of services for adolescents.

The reasons for the underuse of services by impaired youth as well as the underrecognition by health care professionals of mental health problems in general health care settings are thought to be many. They are beyond the scope of this discussion with the exception of one critical factor: the role of health professionals' attitudes, skills, and knowledge of psychological and behavioral aspects and the impact this knowledge or its lack may have on the identification of at-risk youth and their treatment and continuity of care. Several studies suggest that the lack of training of physicians in communication skills, behavioral issues, and knowledge and attitudes about mental health treatments and community resources are crucial factors in how these issues are handled in the health care setting (Fletcher 1980; Goldberg 1984). In turn, this will influence the perception by youth and their families about the appropriateness of the health care setting for seeking help for mental health problems (Hickson et al. 1983).

A U.S. Department of Health and Human Services (1989a) report suggests that during the past 10 years, health professions schools (e.g., schools of social work, nursing, psychology, and psychiatry) have expanded their training programs in suicide prevention. It is clear, however, that the scope of these programs varies widely across disciplines, across medical specialties, and across the various programs themselves. A study of a national sample of training programs in the major medical (*nonpsychiatry*) specialties showed that emergency psychiatry training, including the identification and emergent or acute treatment of patients who are suicidal, was "meager" (Weissberg 1990). Most (70%) of the programs *did not* provide formal or systematic instruction in these areas, even at a knowledge-content level (i.e., lectures and seminars).

In a study of physicians in California, 90% reported feeling that their knowledge of suicide was insufficient (Rockwell and O'Brien 1973). More recently, when practicing physicians in various specialties were asked to identify well-known risk factors for suicide in a paper-and-pencil test, an average of 6 of 13 signs were not recognized as such (Burdick et al. 1983).

Examination of the standards for graduate medical education, as described in the *Directory of Graduate Medical Education* (1995–1996), reveals that primary care specialties and others likely to come in contact with suicidal patients, such as family practice, pediatrics, internal medicine, emergency medicine, obstetrics and gynecology, and surgery do not specifically include suicidal risk and its management in their curricula. This is true even though at least 50% of these specialties' training directors endorse the idea that knowledge of emergency psychiatry, including knowledge about suicide, is helpful for the practice of their specialty (Weissberg 1990).

It is questionable whether health care professionals currently obtain this knowledge through continuing education if it is not obtained during residency training. Most likely they do not; this has not been studied in specialties other than mental health. Even in a study of a sample of mental health professionals, fewer than one in four psychiatrists and psychologists in the Washington, D.C., area who average 11 years in independent practice have had any postresidency or graduate school training in suicide assessment (Berman and Cohen-Sandler 1982).

We have discussed issues pertaining to the needs and opportunities in training health care professionals in the front lines, the so-called gatekeepers. The particular training needs of those expected to provide expert care (i.e., mental health professionals), although similar in some respects, require separate attention. Mental health professionals, and especially psychiatrists, are expected to be the experts in suicide care, and other disciplines draw on them for consultation and training. There has been relatively little research done on the current state of the organization and implementation of training in suicide care in general or in adolescence in particular in the mental health professions. What there is suggests that at least in some mental health professions, the specific inclusion of suicide in curricula is limited. For example, Bongar and Harmatz (1991), in a study of postgraduate psychology programs, found that only 40% of all graduate programs in clinical psychology offered formal training in the study of suicide. A more specialized area such as adolescent suicide could be expected to receive even less formal attention.

Training requirements in psychiatry specifically mention suicide (*Directory of Graduate Medical Education* 1995–1996). Current "Special Requirements for Residency Training in Psychiatry" state: "There must be organized instruction and supervised clinical experience in emergency psychiatry that . . . should include the assessment and management of patients who are a danger to themselves or others, the evaluation and reduction of risk to caregivers, and knowledge of relevant issues in forensic psychiatry. There should be sufficient continued contact with patients to enable the resident to evaluate the effectiveness of clinical interventions" (American Medical Association 1995, p. 223). A recent survey (Hillard et al. 1993) of the teaching of emergency psychiatry in general psychiatric training programs found that 100% of those responding to the survey included specific didactic and experiential components in suicidology in their programs; 95% reported including specific instruction also in child and adolescent psychiatric emergencies including suicide. Less is known, however, about the extent and character of these experiences. Interestingly, current child psychiatric training standards do not specifically mention suicide in the training requirements (*Directory of Graduate Medical Education* 1995–1996).

The Report of the Secretary's Task Force on Youth Suicide (U.S. Department of Health and Human Services 1989a), in its recommendations for suicide prevention services, underscores the shortage of mental health professionals trained to deal with the particularities of psychological and behavioral disorders in youth and the need for all mental health disciplines to address this specific need.

General Health Care Training

The development of suicide care training programs for health care professionals requires the identification of a body of knowledge plus appropriate skills and attitudes that are fundamental and specifically relevant to competent practice. Some of the issues that need to be considered within such training programs are listed below.

Knowledge

At a minimum, health professionals should acquire knowledge during training (pre- and postgraduate) about warning signs of suicide; risk factors, including the presence of psychiatric disorders such as affective and conduct disorders, and substance (especially alcohol) abuse; previous psychiatric and suicidal history; environmental risk including family psychiatric disorders, suicidal behaviors, and violence; access to firearms; and health risks such as AIDS and other chronic illnesses. In addition, general knowledge about treatment alternatives and community resources for referral is crucial. Knowledge of normal adolescent development relevant to assessment of risk and symptom presentation is another important component.

Skills

The acquisition of skills in interviewing youth and families, particularly those with a youngster at risk for suicide, should have a high priority among training objectives. In a study of nursing students, Inman et al. (1984) found a low correlation between knowledge of suicide risk factors and suicide interviewing skills; the capacity to work effectively with suicidal patients does not automatically follow from merely knowing the risk factors. In addition, in the hurried environment of a busy clinic or emergency service, health professionals need not only effective communication skills but also other tools such as screening questions that may facilitate communication. For example, several studies have found that providing clinicians in an adolescent medicine clinic or other setting with screening questions on abuse, another sensitive and frequently underdetected condition in medical settings (American Medical Association Council on Scientific Affairs 1993), significantly increased the rate of detection of abuse (Johnson and Sheir 1985; Sorensen and Snow 1991).

Health care professionals are in the position to provide continuing general health care to at-risk youths and their families. They should have skills to promote adaptive individual and family functioning, particularly those functions related to the prevention of suicide, and to recognize risk factors such as depression. Treatment approaches using brief problem-oriented counseling (Hawton et al. 1981), group interventions for enhancing cognitive and problem-solving skills (G. Clarke et al. 1993), and brief cognitive-behavioral family therapy (S. Miller et al. 1992) might be useful as secondary interventions after appropriate consultation and thorough evaluation. In addition, skills in using other professional and community resources appropriately and efficiently should be developed during training.

Attitudes

Many myths about suicide need to be dispelled among health professionals. Common misconceptions such as those that suggest that asking a patient directly about suicide will put the idea into a patient's head, that if a patient talks openly about suicide it indicates he or she will not do it, or that attention-getting gestures can be disregarded as easily distinguishable from serious threats, need to be given particular consideration in a training program. Some of these myths are related to lack of specific knowledge, to common societal attitudes toward suicidal behavior, and to the intense feelings often evoked by these situations. Therefore, an effective training program must include the opportunity to examine common clinician fears such as those of involvement, of incompetence, and of anger (Shein 1976). This is of particular importance in settings where clinicians deal with life-threatening conditions because suicidal youngsters are sometimes thought to be causing their own problems (Adler and Jellinek 1990). There must be opportunity also for discussion of the personal values and reactions of the individual practitioner and the experience of sharing some of these issues with experienced clinicians in his or her own field or with mental health consultants. These activities should foster the development of reflective attitudes in health professionals; they should facilitate awareness of reactions to suicidal patients as well as the knowledge of when it is appropriate and timely to seek consultative help. Most importantly, a training program should foster the development of empathic attitudes and the ability to listen, along with a firm, nonambivalent commitment to life (see Chapter 6).

It is essential that attitudes and knowledge of physicians with respect to the potential efficacy of treatment for suicidal youngsters be a priority (Brodaty et al. 1982; Starfield and Borkowf 1969). In particular, it is important to foster appreciation of the importance of interdisciplinary work. Youngsters at suicidal risk and their families often have multiple, complex needs and elicit strong feelings that may be effectively handled by a well-trained interdisciplinary team.

Mental Health Care Training

The previously outlined basic knowledge, skills, and attitudes required for adequate training of general health professionals are of course also relevant for the training of child and adolescent mental health professionals. A child and adolescent psychiatrist or a psychiatrist with special training in adolescence is additionally expected to acquire expert-level knowledge, not only in all areas of primary and secondary assessment and intervention, but also, and very importantly, in the ongoing treatment of suicidal youth. In addition, particular expertise in postvention issues as well as in education of other health and mental health professionals and the community in general is expected. It is imperative that requirements such as those previously quoted for residency training in general psychiatry be added to those for residency training in child and adolescent psychiatry.

A pilot survey about training issues in suicide during child and adolescent psychiatric training from the perspective of trainees was conducted by the Ginsburg Fellows on the Committee (R. Seidel and W. Bennett). Its purpose was to obtain pilot data through a semistructured survey questionnaire administered by telephone interview to assess the feasibility of future study using these methods and to suggest areas for further reflection and research.

Eighteen trainees from nine programs (private, public, and university-based) in different regions of the United States participated in a telephone interview. The survey included questions on demographics, level of training, expectations about encountering suicidal adolescents, the number of suicidal patients trainees estimated they had seen, roles and settings of their interventions, perception of program support and teaching activities in suicide, emotional responses to suicide completion and attempts, and perceived impact of these experiences on their work and attitudes.

All trainees reported some orientation or specific didactic experience in the area of suicide. The majority reported exposure to lectures on the topic, although there was a wide range in the number of hours devoted to the subject. Only one trainee reported the experience of observing interviews of suicidal adolescents.

An interesting aspect addressed in the survey was the perceived role of the trainee in the care of these adolescents. The majority of trainees described their main role with suicidal patients as administrative within inpatient wards or as emergency psychiatrist. Only two listed psychotherapy as one of the main roles in their encounters with suicidal adolescents. The number of patients seen for attempted suicide and with serious attempts was highly variable. Only one trainee reported having had a patient who completed suicide.

One-third of the residents reported experiencing some distress related to the management of their cases, including insomnia, the wish to escape, and thoughts of quitting their training; one experienced a ventricular dysrhythmia. They also described an impact on their subsequent handling of cases: for example, half said they were fearful of their next case. The majority, however, also reported that the experiences affected their training positively. They became more comfortable with these situations and more sensitive to important issues in management, such as family, culture, interdisciplinary work, and the need for careful assessment; they read more and requested more didactics in their program.

Residents found programs moderately helpful in dealing with assessment, management of family and community matters, and some of their personal responses. However, they perceived their programs as offering less support in dealing with problems relating to the adolescents' schools, with legal matters, and in addressing their own feelings of isolation and guilt related to their experiences in suicide care. The most effective support was felt to come from some of the individual supervisors.

As noted above, the intent of this small survey was not to draw conclusions about the current status of suicidology training in child and adolescent psychiatry programs. Rather, the pilot data obtained are suggestive of issues and parameters for the development of curricula for suicidology in child and adolescent psychiatry and in other mental health disciplines where particular expertise in working with adolescents is desired.

Recommendations for the Development of Curricula in Adolescent Suicide Care

The studies discussed previously suggest there is a great need for systematic training of gatekeepers in the health care system in the identification and care of suicidal adolescents. Minimal standards of competence, or at least of curricular exposure, should be established in each specialty or discipline according to its specific roles in the care of adolescents. Training programs should implement these standards, and credentialing should be contingent on adequate compliance.

The mental health professions have, of course, a most important role in the promotion of training for other health professionals. Concerted efforts at increasing the level of participation in professional associations, training, accreditation, and standard-setting agencies are needed. An important day-to-day opportunity lies in the use of consultation-liaison services. Peterson and Bongar (1990) have described the opportunity inherent in these services for education of non-psychiatric physicians in knowledge and skills crucial for the care of suicidal patients.

Curricular design for training of professionals in adolescent suicide care must address the following issues.

- *The minimal curricular didactic exposure necessary for competency at each expected level of intervention and for the particularities of the roles of each discipline.* There seems to be tremendous variability across disciplines, medical specialties, and among programs in didactic exposure to suicidology during training. In some cases, exposure seems to be limited or nonexistent. Mental health disciplines, health professions, and specialties within these need to establish the minimum didactic exposure required for basic competency in this area.
- *The teaching methods and clinical experiences necessary for the acquisition of specific skills.* The previously cited study by Inman et al. (1984) supports the notion that knowledge of factors associated with suicide potential and the capacity to respond verbally to individuals at risk for suicide are two independent competency areas. The importance of direct patient care in the development of clinical skills

in both communication and clinical management is generally recognized. However, increasing skill levels often are expected to occur essentially through the handling of high patient loads. One of
residents' main concerns in the survey by Hillard et al. (1993) of
emergency psychiatric training was the high and growing number
of patients for evaluation and management. Much less emphasis
seems to be placed on direct on-site supervision and modeling of
skills. Lomax (1986), in his proposed curriculum on suicide for
general psychiatry residency, recommended that residents be observed firsthand as they evaluate patients and initiate treatment.
He argues for the need to assess specific skills, such as how the trainee
engages the suicidal patient in the interview process, how the trainee
frames questions and responses to facilitate communication, and
how the trainee balances the need to obtain uncomfortable information with the avoidance of undue narcissistic injury to the patient.
Although a trainee in adolescent suicide probably already has considerable experience with suicidal adults, the particularities intro-
duced by developmental considerations justify a similar training
methodology in child and adolescent psychiatric training.

A broader and perhaps more troubling issue is that many training programs currently put little or no emphasis on training residents to perform any kind of psychotherapy, much less the often
more demanding skills required for treating adolescents. Furthermore, insurance companies are generally resistant to paying for
the amount of psychotherapy that might be necessary.

Curricula for the training of professionals in other mental health
and general health care disciplines and subspecialties should include similarly specific clinical, directly supervised experiences appropriate to their expected roles in suicide care.

- *The variety of roles needed to ensure development of the broad range of
skills expected of experts in adolescent suicide care such as child and adolescent psychiatrists.* As noted before, mental health professionals
with particular expertise in adolescence, such as child and adolescent psychiatrists, are expected to acquire expert-level knowledge
in all areas of adolescent suicide care. This knowledge includes
managing early and acute care as well as ongoing treatment and
educating other health and mental health professionals and the
community. Residents responding to our survey indicated that they
had received inadequate support from their programs on issues
such as dealing with schools or courts in relation to their suicidal
patients. In addition, the great majority saw their principal role

vis à vis their patients as administrative (for example, within inpatient services) or in the context of being the emergency department psychiatrist. A balance of roles is necessary so that trainees develop skills not only in acute management and crisis interventions, but also in prevention, long-term treatment, and interventions in the community.

- *The learning experiences specifically needed to facilitate the development of appropriate attitudes.* It is necessary to assess and monitor the development of attitudes in trainees, particularly the development of a reflective attitude—the disposition to and competence in examining and discussing personal responses and concerns about care of suicidal patients. Lomax (1986) suggests that one objective should be that trainees be sufficiently aware of personal difficulties in dealing with suicidal individuals, either to work to overcome them or to know when to refer suicidal patients to those more able to deal with them effectively. Clinicians should be able to evaluate their own personal and technical competencies in working with suicidal patients, and this must be an important aspect of training. Training programs need to consider specifically the curricular elements that will best foster the development of these attitudes, including formal didactics, clinical and personal experiences, and role models.

- *The characteristics of training environments effective in facilitating learning about and coping with emotional responses elicited by work with suicidal patients and, in particular, with the unfortunate event of a patient's suicide.* Therapists consider suicidal behavior one of the most stressful aspects of their work (Deutsch 1984). A survey of a national sample of psychologists and psychiatrists found that 22% of psychologists and 51% of psychiatrists reported having experienced the loss of a patient to suicide (Chemtob et al. 1988b). A few studies have addressed the occurrence of patient suicide during training (H. N. Brown 1987b; Goldstein and Buongiorno 1984; Kahne 1968). H. N. Brown (1987b) suggested that this experience may be more common than generally recognized. In Brown's study, 37% of those psychiatrists surveyed (as well as 14% of psychologists and social workers) had experienced a patient's suicide while in training. The impact of suicide on therapists is considerable (H. N. Brown 1987b; Chemtob et al. 1988a). The experience during training may have an even more powerful impact. Although in the small sample we surveyed only one resident had this experience, the trainees reported that working with seriously suicidal patients had a considerable emotional impact and was associated with a variety of symptoms including sleep disturbances, somatic symptoms, and thoughts of escape or of quitting. Although the handling and working through of feelings of isolation and guilt often elicited by these situations seem to be of special importance for patient care as well as for the trainees' professional development and well-being, as noted in the pilot survey, trainees in some child and adolescent psychiatry programs perceived relatively little support in this area. Programs must identify the kinds of formal activities and characteristics of the program environment that actively support and foster learning of effective coping. For example, activities that permit the sharing and working through of feelings, such as "psychological autopsy" conferences, where trainees and staff, particularly those who have experienced the death of a patient by suicide, can have a meaningful discussion of family survivors' responses and those of caregivers, should be encouraged. In addition, individual and group supervisions should regularly initiate discussions about caregivers' reactions to suicidal patients in those settings where patients are most commonly seen.

- *The qualifications of teachers and supervisors in this area.* In the pilot survey previously discussed, individual supervisors were considered to be the most helpful of all the elements of the program in dealing with trainees' feelings and reactions related to clinical work with suicidal patients. However, as was to be expected, not all supervisors were thought to be helpful or receptive to such work. Lomax (1986), addressing the teaching of suicidology in general psychiatric residency programs, suggests that teachers and supervisors should be individuals with both adequate bases of experience in suicide care and also the personal qualities to enable them to articulate the emotionally charged issues of this topic. Training programs in the different disciplines need to establish the particular qualifications required of effective, supportive supervisors for this kind of work.

Conclusion

Research has already demonstrated many of the training needs for child and adolescent mental health professionals who will be in the role of evaluating and intervening with patients along the continuum of risk for suicide. There is also great need to investigate the kinds of training requirements, experiences, teaching methods, and faculty that will best foster the development of competent, sensitive, and committed caregivers for adolescents at suicidal risk. The studies reviewed here and accumulated experience in the field suggest a number of elements necessary for successful training of a variety of professionals as caregivers for adolescents at suicidal risk. First, there is a need for more specific training requirements in the area of suicide for all health and mental health disciplines and medical specialties involved in the care of adolescents. Second, programs' goals and objectives in this area must be clear for both faculty and trainees. These goals and objectives need to address the development of not only knowledge, but also the skills and attitudes necessary to function effectively at all stages, including prevention, intervention, and postvention. Third, a variety of didactic, clinical, personal, and community experiences must be offered. The development of different competencies requires a variety of approaches and experiences and should occur within the context of programs supportive of trainees' personal growth and well-being. Fourth, professional and credentialing bodies will need to establish minimum criteria for exposure and development of competencies during training in each of the health and mental health disciplines according to their particular roles in the care of adolescents. Finally, there is the crucial need to provide, without fail, professional and peer support for trainees who experience patient suicides or suicide attempts.

8

Medicolegal and Public Policy Aspects of Therapeutic Care

Legal Considerations

The rights of children and adolescents committed to mental institutions are determined by individual states and not by federal constitutional laws. In most states, children younger than 13 or 14 can be admitted by their parents, but once hospitalized, adolescents have the right to seek their own counsel and are entitled to a court hearing to determine the need for involuntary hospitalization. In all states, some provisions exist for involuntary hospitalization by qualified physicians in lieu of parents, but the court can rescind the order as illustrated, unfortunately, by the following vignette.

A 17-year-old depressed female was admitted after an overdose. The patient was initially admitted to the schizophrenia unit because there were no beds on the adolescent unit. The patient's family became upset about this arrangement and demanded and got the patient discharged. They reported that they had had negative past experiences with psychiatrists during treatment of three other family members for bipolar disorder. The patient was subsequently hospitalized involuntarily. The family then hired a lawyer who had the commitment rescinded. The patient shot and killed herself 2 weeks later.

The death of a youth through suicide is a tragedy for the youth, the family, and society. The family is left not only to grieve but also to contend with inevitable feelings of self-recrimination. Right or wrong, a pervasive preoccupation with the whys and wherefores of the suicide afflicts the survivors including any mental health professionals who may have been involved in the treatment of the young person.

Beyond the emotional impact of a suicide, an uncommon but serious consequence for a therapist or a hospital is a liability suit or malpractice action. These are risks that even the most competent mental health professionals and institutions run in such cases. This section reviews the principles of good psychiatric care that, when they are not followed, form the bases for most such actions.

In general, liability exists when a proper standard of care was not provided and the court determines that this factor was a proximate cause of the suicide. An error in judgment on the part of the clinician does not per se constitute sufficient basis for a finding of liability. The court recognizes that clinicians are not reliably able to predict future behavior of their patients and that good psychiatric care requires taking certain risks. For example, there is no expectation that a patient will be hospitalized simply because he or she reveals suicidal ideation. Treatment in the least restrictive setting is generally accepted as a cardinal principle of good psychiatric practice. The errors in good professional practice and management of a case likely to expose the psychiatrist to suit include the following:

- *Failure to do an appropriate, thorough diagnostic evaluation, particularly with regard to suicide potential, including obtaining prior records and a careful family history.* The evaluation would include a thorough exploration of the suicide risk factors (Chapter 3), including the nature of the suicide attempt, the social environment, the demographics (Nurcome 1991), and the physical and psychological factors. When at all possible, family members should be interviewed directly.
- *Failure to hospitalize the patient when the risk appears to warrant this move.* The evaluator must determine whether the home environment is protective and whether the adolescent can feel safe at home under the present circumstances. If there is any doubt whatsoever, hospitalization is the course to follow.

A 15-year-old female was brought to the emergency room by her mother and grandmother who both stated that the patient had threatened to stab herself. The patient reported that she had been using phencyclidine (PCP) and marijuana for approximately 2 weeks and that her mother had just learned about this. During the interview, the mother was judgmental and rejecting, stating that she refused to have her daughter living at home with her under these circumstances. The patient denied any ongoing suicide ideation and stated that she had told her mother that she might as well be dead during a heated argument about her drug use. She denied any intention of harming herself and denied any threats to stab herself. Mother and grandmother refused to take the patient home with them stating that they wanted her admitted to the hospital for evaluation and drug rehabilitation. The patient refused hospitalization; however, the mother demanded admission. Because the patient was a minor, the mother was able to sign the consent forms. The patient became uncooperative, combative, and verbally abusive. She required four-point restraints for transport to the psychiatric unit.

(Under different conditions, involuntary hospitalization may not have been the ideal solution for this youngster. However, in the absence of other safe placement availability, the mother's right to sign the daughter in determined the immediate disposition.)

- *Failure to take adequate protective measures when there is any likelihood of suicide.* The therapist must provide appropriate suicide precautions such as removing all agents capable of causing death from the patient's access and institute appropriate suicide observation procedures and nursing care.
- *Failure to provide specific written orders and to communicate clearly all relevant decisions to the support staff and failure to keep a clearly documented record.* Written orders must be very specific; it is not enough to order "suicide precautions." Should observation be constant or every 15 minutes? Should the patient have a full-time, one-on-one coverage? The rationale for all medication or treatment initiatives should be noted. Staff should be asked to note particular signs, symptoms, or behavior that the treating psychiatrist thinks may indicate the patient's mental condition. Staff notes should be read daily and discussions held as needed. A physician could be considered negligent if he or she gave a verbal order for one-on-one observation but did not document the reasons for doing so. Nurse and staff observations of the patient's mood and behavior as well as the adolescent's overheard comments are extremely important to document. The reasons whether or not to continue suicidal precautions should be stated in writing.

Adequate record keeping is a clinician's best protection against loss of a malpractice suit. Anything not recorded is assumed not to have happened. All significant information and other communications should be noted, whether the source is the patient, family, or hospital staff.

- *Failure to involve the family and to maintain open communication in both directions.* The family evaluation is important before discharge can be contemplated. Failure to assess the home setting as previously noted could constitute malpractice. When the family is available, every effort should be made by the therapist to involve the family as partners in the decisions regarding the care of the patient. If there is the suicide of a minor, it will be the family that is plaintiff in a liability action. The quality of the relationship that the youth's therapist has maintained with the family may be a significant factor in whether or not a suit is lodged.

- *Failure to maintain life-sustaining hospitalization for the adolescent (premature discharge must be avoided).* Many hospitals are threatened by insurance companies and managed care corporations with having reimbursement discontinued if patients remain hospitalized for an "unnecessary" length of time. It is important to keep the suicidal patient in a protective environment as long as deemed necessary by the *clinical* staff and not to succumb to administrative pressures that are decidedly not in the patient's best interests.

It is essential that the clinician dealing with a nonhospitalized suicidal patient be available 24 hours per day to both the adolescent and to the family. If the issue of whether to hospitalize or not arises, the clinician is well-advised to hold a family meeting in which a risk-benefit analysis of such a move is carefully laid out and the family encouraged to express their wishes. If the therapist's inclination is to risk outpatient treatment rather than choose the safer course of hospitalizing the youth, the family will support that choice in most cases. The family that has felt included or was consulted in such important decisions is less likely to turn on the treating psychiatrist if a tragedy ensues.

When the adolescent is hospitalized, the clinician must keep in mind a number of considerations. For a voluntary admission, the patient may be free to come and go (an unwise degree of freedom if suicide is a serious risk). The patient should be seen as soon as possible after admission by the treating psychiatrist, generally within a few hours. If a suicide gesture or attempt has occurred or if suicide preoccupations are persistent, the therapist must recognize that an emergency situation exists. At that point, the usual constraining rules of confidentiality no longer apply. This is fully recognized by the American Psychiatric Association in its ethical guidelines. The clinician who chooses to work alone rather than enlisting the help of the family at such a time creates an unnecessary handicap. At the same time, he or she is increasing the likelihood of unwelcome legal repercussions in the event of a completed suicide.

Therapist anxiety in suicidal situations is unavoidable and can, of course, get in the way of effective treatment. Paying careful attention to minimizing the legal risks has the additional benefit of lessening the clinician's anxiety and may render therapeutic efforts more effective.

Public Considerations

Because suicide is a leading cause of death for adolescents, as well as an often preventable one, it is appropriate to consider it as a public health problem. As we have seen in earlier chapters, some of the risk factors for adolescent suicide are rooted in social ills, such as poverty, that are beyond the scope of psychiatric interventions. Others, such as depression and substance abuse, can be effectively addressed through early identification and appropriate interventions. Public policy initiatives can focus on enhancing recognition of depression and other risk factors, as well as improving treatment. Targeted research funding can address the need to increase our knowledge about vulnerability and risk factors, as well as outcomes of interventions.

Numerous groups and organizations concerned with the mental health needs of children and youth have called for a national mandate to address the problems of unmet needs, citing the increasing rates of adolescent suicide as one consequence of failure to address inadequate mental health care for children and adolescents. Increasing mental health care and treatment for adolescents is one of the most often repeated policy recommendations. Psychiatrists, because of their expertise in providing direct care to suicidal adolescents, have much to offer in helping to shape public policy through consultation and education in their local communities, as well as through serving as policy advisors to state and national government agencies. Indeed, the influence of psychiatrists knowledgeable about adolescent suicide has already been felt through the initiatives described below. However, much remains to be done.

In 1969 the Joint Commission on Mental Health of Children stated that 85% of children and adolescents identified as having emotional problems and learning disorders were not seen by any mental health professional (Joint Commission on Mental Health of Children 1969); the United States Congress, Office of Technology Assessment (U.S. Congress, OTA 1991) report estimated this at about 70% in 1986. J. L. Rubinstein et al. (1989) found that 60 students of 300 "normal" adolescents surveyed, not identified as having psychiatric problems, admitted to suicidal behavior; 45 of these suicidal adolescents had received no therapeutic intervention in the year in which the suicidal behavior took place, despite having a similar psychological profile to hospitalized suicidal adolescents, which demonstrates great inconsistency in handling suicidal adolescents.

Improved access to mental health treatment for adolescents is vital. A recent report on private office visits to psychiatrists showed that only 5% of these visits were by patients under age 15 and 7.9% by patients age 15–24 (Shuppert 1993). If we attempt to extrapolate from these figures to the 12–18 age group, it is likely that only 6%–7% of visits were by this age group or about 3 per 100 persons. Given the conservatively estimated prevalence of serious mental disorders in adolescents of 5%–6%, this figure is clearly low. These figures lend support to the general agreement that access to health care, including mental health care, is inadequate for adolescents, perhaps more so than for any other age group. The recent publicity surrounding what appears to have been excessive use of psychiatric hospitalization for adolescents in some communities should not obscure the fact that most adolescents in need of mental health services never receive them.

At the request of numerous members of Congress, the OTA studied the physical, emotional, and behavioral health of contemporary American adolescents. In 1991, the OTA published a three-volume work, *Adolescent Health* (U.S. Congress, OTA 1991), which includes the findings of the study and policy recommendations. This document notes that adolescent suicide rates have increased in recent years and that adolescents with mental health or substance abuse problems, concerns about sexual identity, school problems, family disruption and parental loss, loss of a close friend, or exposure to other adolescent suicides are all at increased risk. Policy recommendations to increase mental health services to adolescents include expanding insurance coverage for both inpatient and outpatient care; educating adolescents about when and how to seek mental health services; and supporting the development of more accessible, comprehensive, and appropriate services. Examples cited of such services are "wrap-around services"[1] and services in school settings for adolescents who do not yet have a diagnosable mental disorder. Better training for mental health providers on treating adolescents is advocated. A parallel set of recommendations in the same work deals with funding for research on services and psychiatric disorders.

The Institute of Medicine of the National Academy of Sciences (1989) reported on the current state of research-based knowledge about child and adolescent mental disorders. The report noted that rates of substance abuse, homicide, and suicide were escalating among disadvantaged children and youth and pointed out the need to discover risk as well as protective factors. This group also pointed out the importance of follow-up studies and stated, "Currently there are no mechanisms to support the needed programmatic research" to allow for follow-up of patients 1 to 2 years posttreatment to evaluate treatment outcomes. Other specific research goals relevant to adolescent suicide included "how primary care providers recognize, diagnose, and treat mental illness in children and adolescents," and "the possible reduction of subsequent drug abuse by early treatment of depression or anxiety disorders."

More research is needed to understand fully the risk factors involved in adolescent suicide and to properly evaluate prevention activities. A special Task Force on Youth Suicide (U.S. Department of Health and Human Services 1989a, 1989b) convened by the Secretary of Health and Human Services reviewed the current body of knowledge on adolescent suicide and published a four-volume report in 1989. The report decried the dearth of research specifically on adolescents and made six recommendations: 1) better data on suicide and suicide attempts, 2) research on risk factors, 3) research on effectiveness and cost of interventions to prevent suicide, 4) support for suicide prevention services,

---

[1]Wrap-around services are an array of services developed to meet the needs of youngsters who would otherwise be in institutional placements. Services are tailored to the needs of individual children and adolescents based on an assessment by a behavioral specialist. These services typically include in-home supervision by a mental health worker sometimes on a 24-hour basis. Family therapy may be provided via home visits by a family therapist if the family does not have transportation, and transportation for medical follow-up is arranged. An intensive case manager is assigned to coordinate services. Although these services are typically provided to children and adolescents with long-term mental illnesses after other less intensive forms of treatment have failed or after multiple hospitalizations, they may be appropriate for chronically depressed youngsters who are at risk for multiple suicide attempts.

5) education of the public and health service providers, and 6) involvement of both the public and private sectors in prevention activities. In accordance with the task force's recommendations, research funding was increased. Treatment intervention research projects have been funded that focus on improving life skills, problem solving, mood management, and social networks in high-risk teenagers and young adults in high school, college, and military settings.

The federal government has undertaken several steps to respond to suicide, including adolescent suicide, as a public health problem. The National Institute of Mental Health (NIMH) has targeted the prevention of suicidal behavior as one of its priorities, and NIMH awards grants for research and clinical training in this area through its Prevention Research Branch and Division of Clinical Research, respectively. One of NIMH's initiatives, the Depression/Awareness, Recognition, and Treatment Program, is a public education program focused on primary health care providers, mental health clinicians, and the general public. Its goal is to increase recognition and treatment of depression.

Despite such efforts, federal funding for initiatives that would address the problem of adolescent suicide remains low. Funding for the Child Mental Health Services Program, a federal grant program, was reduced from the $100 million per year originally proposed to $4.9 million for fiscal year 1993.

Recent amendments to the State Comprehensive Mental Health Services Plan Act, a federal law that deals with funding to states for mental health, require that studies be done related to the care of children with serious emotional problems under the provisions of Public Law 94-142. This is an example of a mechanism by which the federal initiatives can influence the direction of services and research on the state and local level without necessarily involving increased expenditures of funds. Federal directives not withstanding, numerous initiatives do exist on the state and local level, although information about them is not widely available. The state of Maryland, for example, has an Office of Suicide Prevention that provides training for mental health professionals and school personnel. Some have argued that efforts regarding health and welfare are best left to the states (Haggerty 1991) because the Constitution delegates health affairs to the states and because the states have greater flexibility to adapt to regional needs.

Physicians, through their professional organizations, have acted on their concerns about adolescent suicide by working to improve the quality and accessibility of care for high risk adolescents. *Child and Adolescent Psychiatry: Guidelines for Treatment Resources, Quality Assurance, Peer*

Review and Reimbursement (Stevenson and Maholick 1987) was an attempt by the American Academy of Child and Adolescent Psychiatry to address the controversy over psychiatric hospitalization of adolescents by setting forth standards for hospitalization. Because suicidality is an important reason for hospitalization of adolescents, these recommendations are particularly applicable to the suicidal adolescent. The document pointed out that the presence of a psychiatric diagnosis or symptoms was not sufficient reason for hospitalization, but rather the level of impairment in functioning and need for a comprehensive treatment program were.

In addition to advocating for careful psychiatric assessment before the decision for hospitalization, the authors stated that intensive treatment programs for children and adolescents should be under the direction of psychiatrists who are trained to care for these patient age groups. The document differentiated between acute hospital programs, which primarily evaluate, stabilize, and provide brief treatment, and intermediate and long-term inpatient psychiatric treatment programs, with intermediate programs lasting 3–15 months and long-term care ranging from 12 to 48 months. The latter are necessary for patients whose "disabilities are longstanding and progressive despite intensive efforts to conduct treatment in less intensive settings" (Stevenson and Maholick 1987, p. 3). This kind of intensive treatment requires sufficient time for the remediation of multiple deficits. The importance of continuity of care was stressed.

Improved case-finding and better treatment by primary care providers are important aspects of prevention of adolescent suicide. The importance of primary care providers as a resource for adolescents with emotional problems is underscored by several studies. Between 50% and 60% of all diagnosed mental disorders are treated by nonpsychiatric providers. An estimated 15%–30% of patients seen in primary care settings have a currently diagnosable mental illness with frequencies of medical use at least twice those of comparable populations without these problems (Jacobsen et al. 1980). However, the physicians who see these high-risk youngsters do not usually address their psychiatric needs.

Obviously, appropriate care can only be provided if a problem is recognized, and depression is one of the most frequently missed diagnoses in primary care settings. Unfortunately, adolescents rarely turn to primary care physicians for help with emotional distress, and physicians do not routinely screen for emotional disorders. Thus one likely avenue to mental health services for those in need is greatly underused. One reason for this is lack of ability of these physicians to do a diagnostic assessment of the patients they see. A corollary is that their adolescent patients do not see their doctors as a resource. Training for pediatricians, family practice specialists, and internists in the diagnosis and treatment of common adolescent psychiatric disorders is important, but equally important is the opportunity for consultation with a psychiatrist who can assist the primary care physician in evaluating suicide risk in adolescent patients and in obtaining appropriate services for these patients. Much remains to be done before primary care physicians can be considered an effective resource for the prevention of adolescent suicide.

The American Academy of Pediatrics has recognized the need for pediatricians to be knowledgeable about adolescent suicide, including it in its training modules for recertification, and training in psychosocial issues is a required part of pediatric residency training. The American Academy of Pediatrics has recommended that pediatricians routinely screen for a variety of psychosocial problems when they see adolescent patients and has offered specific guidelines for such screening (American Academy of Pediatrics 1988). As we have discussed, adolescents with mental disorders including adolescents contemplating suicide are more likely to be seen by primary care providers than by psychiatrists, so that primary care providers represent a potentially important source of care for these youngsters. These providers could be involved in three ways, by early diagnosis, by assessment and triage, and by appropriate follow-up care either by the primary care physician or through referral to a specialist.

The American Medical Association has developed a series of guidelines for primary care physicians to provide preventive services to adolescents. These guidelines recommend that adolescents be seen on a yearly basis, be screened for a variety of problems, and be given health education, counseling, and anticipatory guidance. The guidelines state, "All adolescents should be asked annually about behaviors or emotions that indicate recurrent or severe depression or risk of suicide." Psychiatric referral is recommend for suspected suicide risk or symptoms of severe or recurrent depression (American Medical Association 1995; Elster and Kuznets 1993).

Access to therapeutic care is limited by lack of availability, including physical location, hours, and "user-friendliness" of services and by lack of insurance coverage. School-based services are recognized as greatly diminishing physical and psychological barriers to use (Dryfoos 1991). Obviously, expansion of insurance coverage to include adolescents' outpatient visits to organized mental health services is essential, as only half of these visits are currently covered (U.S. Congress, OTA 1991).

Only half of the states now have statutes that allow adolescents to obtain mental health treatment on their own with various restrictions. A limitation of access to mental health treatment is imposed by restrictions on adolescents' ability to obtain services without parental consent, although in most cases they may obtain treatment for substance abuse, sexually transmitted diseases, and pregnancy. The Committee on Adolescence believes strongly that parents should be involved in the adolescents' decision to seek treatment and that their knowledge of, support of, and frequently, active involvement in the ongoing treatment is important. At the same time, the committee recognizes that for some suicidal adolescents the possibility of seeking treatment and entering into a therapeutic relationship on their own would greatly facilitate their obtaining essential and timely intervention. Available research, as well as knowledge about adolescent cognitive development, supports the idea that adolescents are capable of giving informed consent to health care including mental health services. The enactment of legislation that would allow this to occur in cases where adolescents are deemed at risk for self-harm is strongly supported.

The suicide rate for juveniles in jail is five times higher than the national average and the first few hours of confinement are the most dangerous (U.S. Department of Health and Human Services 1989a). Among homeless and runaway teenagers, rates of depression, suicide attempts, and suicidal ideation are all high. Studies have found up to half of these adolescents to have histories of previous suicide attempts. Adolescents such as these, who are at risk for suicide, may not be seen by medical personnel at all but do come in contact with various social agencies. As such they are likely to be seen by social workers, probation officers, the family court staff, or school personnel. Policies for early identification and intervention education should be implemented for social, health, and educational agencies.

Few programs that involve mental health promotion efforts targeted to adolescents have been implemented, although these programs are another component of suicide prevention. Although specific suicide prevention programs in schools and communities may not be effective in achieving their goals of dissuading adolescents from suicide, more broadly based programs aimed at increasing awareness that psychiatric disorders are prevalent and treatable and at reducing the stigma attached to seeking mental health services can indirectly help by increasing the likelihood that troubled adolescents will seek help. Mental health promotion programs can be defined as nonspecific efforts to improve mental and emotional stability as opposed to specific efforts to prevent a certain type of disorder (much as good nutrition to promote physical health compares with measles vaccinations). These kinds of general programs improve coping skills and social and academic performance. Although their usefulness in preventing adolescent suicide has not been systematically studied, the good outcomes that have been shown from these programs make them highly desirable. These programs can generally be conducted by school personnel who are given training to run them and incorporated easily into the school setting, which makes them potentially cost-effective. When one thinks of the amount of funding expended on the recent revision of nutritional recommendations to be taught in classrooms, the cost of these programs would be insignificant.

Firearms are implicated in a large percentage of completed suicides. Although guns do not cause suicidal ideation and impulses, the ready availability of guns may increase the likelihood that an impulsive youngster will use them as a means of self-destruction, and if guns are used, the effect is likely to be lethal. Effective control of firearms must be attained. The Task Force on Youth Suicide (U.S. Department of Health and Human Services 1989a) made several recommendations regarding firearms, including better enforcement of laws, limitations on advertising (especially to young people), improvement in safety features of guns, gun safety education, and research to evaluate gun control programs. The American Medical Association has recommended that primary care physicians counsel families of adolescents to avoid having firearms in the home if possible, to make them inaccessible to adolescents if they are in the home, and to ensure that adolescents follow safety procedures if they do have weapons (American Medical Association 1995).

There have been many calls to action and too few responses. Opportunities for having an impact on the preventable tragedy of adolescent suicide exist on all levels from the federal government to the local community as well as in individual offices and clinics. Psychiatrists can play a major role through their activities in their professional organizations as well as through political action and can be crucial in educating the public as well as their professional colleagues about what can be done to help the suicidal adolescent and about the importance of suicide prevention efforts.

9

Summary and Conclusions

In the introduction to this report our committee, with its focus on adolescent development, expressed its concern that adolescent suicidal behavior represented a grave crisis in the adolescent, a crisis not only in the development of the adolescent but one that endangers the existence of the adolescent. The possibility of a fatal outcome is abhorrent to us as physicians and psychiatrists, as it is to all those entrusted with the care and development of our fellow human beings. Consequently, we explored the ways in which developmental and other forces lead to adolescent suicide and the measures that can be taken to prevent it.

We first considered the historical and cross-cultural aspects of suicidal behaviors. Societal and cultural stresses arise from parental attitudes, beliefs, expectations, and childrearing practices that evolve from the social and economic needs in each culture. If unbalanced by growth-sustaining supports, they may compromise or constrict the existential adaptive ability of the developing adolescent and place the adolescent at risk for suicide.

Research into vulnerability in adolescence has revealed gender, ethnic, and geographic differences in the dimension of the problem and has indicated the social, psychological, and biological conditions that increase the likelihood that adolescents will resort to suicidal behaviors. Research is still needed to distinguish those adolescents who commit suicide from those adolescents with similar conditions who do not. Research has only begun to explore the ways in which the interaction of specific individual dynamics, precipitating events, and personal characteristics result in an adolescent's attempt of suicide.

We discussed the strengths that adolescents acquire, but we emphasized the weaknesses that ensue as adolescents are faced with the impact of the thrust of their own biological, psychological, and social development with the forces inherent in their cultures. Adolescents progress through this period in their lives with varying and varied attempts to master, or cope with, the inevitable change in their existential status. Some try but fail and some fail to try, with resulting despair that can lead those adolescents to believe that suicide is the only choice they have to end their suffering.

We described how psychodynamics can influence motivation, relationships, and behaviors, and how these may contribute to an outcome of suicide. Existing psychopathological conditions contribute. These include anxiety, dysthymia, posttraumatic stress disorders, acute reactive disorders, major affective disorders, severe conduct disorders, and psychotic disorders. We considered the possible lethal interplay between psychodynamic and psychopathological factors.

This led to the crux of this report, a full discussion of prevention and treatment. The first and most important aspect of suicide prevention is early recognition of the adolescent at risk. It is of high priority to detect and treat those psychiatric disorders accompanied by greatest suicidal risk: depression, conduct disorders, substance abuse disorders, borderline conditions, and schizoaffective disorders. With all adolescents, threats of suicide must be taken seriously. There should be an immediate, complete psychiatric workup preferably before specific treatment begins. If crisis intervention must precede diagnostic study, the workup should not be delayed longer than necessary. Education of health care professionals, educators, families, and peers about warning signs can emphasize early intervention and thereby enable a skilled psychiatrist to assess suicidal thoughts, plans, means, and previous attempts, past and current life stresses, and available family and environmental support. All of this information will lead to a decision regarding hospitalization and treatment for the adolescent.

Treatment includes a careful diagnosis of all accompanying disorders; an ongoing assessment of suicidal risk; an evaluation of the adolescent's interpersonal skills and adaptive strengths; an awareness of the patient's attitudes, emotions, and expectations toward the therapist; and a recognition by the therapist of his or her own responses to the suicidal adolescent. Therapeutic modalities include short-term individual psychotherapy focused on problem solving and support; cognitive therapy; peer group therapy; family therapy; use of a network of therapists, teachers, counselors, agencies, clergy, and probation officers;

establishment of a safety contract and safety watch; long-term residential treatment; psychopharmacological treatment for specific disorders; and long-term psychoanalytic psychotherapy. In the event that an adolescent completes a suicide, a therapist working with family, friends, teachers, peers, and the adolescent's therapist and therapeutic team, if there was one, may help relieve possible feelings such as helplessness, guilt, and isolation.

The goals of prevention, early identification, management, and treatment of suicidal behavior can be attained only through the efforts of responsible caregivers who are adequately trained. There is a present need to develop the requisite knowledge, skills, and attitudes in all who come in responsible contact with potentially suicidal youth, especially general health and mental health professionals. Training methods include didactic instruction, firsthand observation, supervised experience, demonstration of the various roles that caregivers must assume, exploration of attitudes, and encouragement of consultation with colleagues.

In the event of a completed suicide, an uncommon but serious reaction by the family to the emotional impact is a liability suit or malpractice action. The best professional protection also is the best professional practice. This includes a thorough diagnostic evaluation, hospitalization when the risk warrants it, provision of suicidal precautions in hospital, making thoroughly understood specific written orders to staff, frequent contact with the patient, open and fully available communication with the family, maintenance of hospitalization for as long as necessary, and institution of responsible follow-up care.

In the broadest sense, it is important to consider adolescent suicidal behavior as a public health problem, which must call on public and private funding of mental health services, education, training, and research related to intervention and prevention.

Suicidal behavior in adolescents does not represent a single syndrome or psychopathological entity. The risk of suicide results from the interplay of a multiplicity of biological, psychological, and sociocultural factors. To provide effective prevention, early detection, and treatment, it is necessary to implement the broad range of interventions that we have discussed. This is essential for all potentially suicidal adolescents, including those who have suicidal thoughts, those who make threats and gestures, and those who make serious and near fatal attempts to kill themselves. All suicidal behavior presents a threat to the lives of our adolescents, and if untreated it remains a threat to their development. Given timely and effective care, suicidal adolescents will be able to adapt to their societies and make their contributions toward progressive challenge and change.

References

Adityanjee: Suicide attempts and suicide in India: cross-cultural aspects. Int J Soc Psychiatry 32:64–73, 1986

Adler R, Jellinek MS: Suicide, in Psychiatric Aspects of General Hospital Pediatrics. Edited by Jellinek MS, Herzog D. Chicago, IL, Year Book Medical, 1990

Akiskal HS, Downs J, Jordan P, et al: Affective disorders in referred children and younger siblings of manic-depressives: mode of onset and prospective course. Arch Gen Psychiatry 42:996–1103, 1985

Ambrosini PJ, Rabinovich H, Puig-Antich J: Biological factors and pharmacologic treatment in major depressive disorder in children and adolescents, in Suicide in the Young. Edited by Sudak HS, Ford AB, Rushford NB. Boston, MA, John Wright, 1984

American Academy of Pediatrics, Committee on Psychosocial Aspects of Child and Family Health: Guidelines for Health Supervision, II. Elk Grove Village, IL, American Academy of Pediatrics, 1988

American Medical Association, Department of Adolescent Health: Guidelines for Adolescent Preventive Services. Chicago, IL, American Medical Association Press, 1992

American Medical Association: The Essentials of Accredited Residencies in Graduate Medical Education. Chicago, IL, American Medical Association Press, 1995

American Medical Association, Council on Scientific Affairs: Adolescents as the victims of family violence. JAMA 270:1850–1856, 1993

American Psychiatric Association: Diagnostic and Statistical Manual of Mental Disorders, 3rd Edition. Washington, DC, American Psychiatric Association, 1980

American Psychiatric Association: Diagnostic and Statistical Manual of Mental Disorders, 3rd Edition, Revised. Washington, DC, American Psychiatric Association, 1987

American Psychiatric Association: Diagnostic and Statistical Manual of Mental Disorders, 4th Edition. Washington, DC, American Psychiatric Association, 1994

Apter A, Bleich A, Plutchik R, et al: Suicidal behavior, depression, and conduct disorder in hospitalized adolescents. J Am Acad Child Adolesc Psychiatry 27:696–699, 1988

Asarnow JR, Carlson GA: Suicide attempts in preadolescent child psychiatry inpatients. Suicide Life Threat Behav 18:129–136, 1988

Asarnow JR, Carlson GA, Guthrie D: Coping strategies, self-perceptions, hopelessness, and perceived family environments in depressed and suicidal children. J Consult Clin Psychol 55:361–366, 1987

Asberg M, Thoren P, Traskman L, et al: Serotonin depression. Science 191:478–480, 1976

Asberg M, Schalling D, Traskman-Benz L, et al: Psychobiology of suicide impulsivity and related phenomena, in Psychopharmacology: The Third Generation of Progress. Edited by Meltzer HY. New York, Raven, 1987

Ballenger JC, Goodwin FK, Major LF, et al: Alcohol and central serotonin metabolism in man. Arch Gen Psychiatry 36:224–227, 1979

Barraclough BM, Bunch J, Nelson B, et al: A hundred cases of suicide. Br J Psychiatry 125:355–373, 1974

Bateson G: Steps to an Ecology of Mind. New York, Ballantine Books, 1972

Beck AT: Cognitive Therapy and the Emotional Disorders. New York, International Universities Press, 1976

Beck AT, Weissman A, Lester D, et al: The measurement of pessimism: the hopelessness scale. J Consult Clin Psychol 42:861–865, 1974

Beck AT, Steer RA, Kovacs M, et al: Hopelessness and eventual suicide. Am J Psychiatry 142:559–563, 1985

Bedrosian RC, Epstein N: Cognitive therapy of depressed and suicidal adolescents, in Suicide in the Young. Edited by Sudak HS, Ford AB, Rushforth NB. London, John Wright, 1984

Berkovitz IH: Elements of optimum suicide prevention climate in schools, in Expanding Mental Health Interventions in Schools. Edited by Berkovitz IH, Seliger JS. Dubuque, IA, Kendall/Hunt, 1985

Berman AL, Cohen-Sandler R: Suicide and the standard of care: optimal vs. acceptable. Suicide Life Threat Behav 12:114–122, 1982

Bertelson A, Harvald B, Hague M: A Danish twin study of manic-depressive disorder. Br J Psychiatry 130:330–351, 1975

Blumenthal SJ, Kupfer DJ: Generalizable treatment strategies for suicidal behavior. Ann N Y Acad Sci 487:327–340, 1986

Bolger N, Downey G, Walker E, et al: The onset of suicide ideation in childhood and adolescence. Journal of Youth and Adolescence 18:175–190, 1989

Bongar B, Harmatz M: Clinical psychology graduate education in the study of suicide: availability, resources, and importance. Suicide Life Threat Behav 21:231–244, 1991

Boor M: Relationship of internal-external control and national suicide rates. J Soc Psychol 100:143–144, 1976

Boor M, Bair JH: Suicide rates, handgun control laws, and sociodemographic variables. Psychol Rep 66:923–930, 1990

Borst SR, Noam GG, Bartok JA: Adolescent suicidality: a clinical-developmental approach. J Am Acad Child Adolesc Psychiatry 30:796–803, 1991

Boyd JH, Moscicki EK: Firearms and youth suicide. Am J Public Health 76:1240–1242, 1986

Brent DA: Over-representation of epileptics among a consecutive series of suicide attempters seen at a children's hospital. Journal of the American Academy of Child Psychiatry 25:242–246, 1986

Brent DA, Perper JA, Allman CJ: Alcohol, firearms and suicide among youth. JAMA 257:3369–3372, 1987

Brent DA, Perper JA, Goldstein CE: Risk factors for adolescent suicide: a comparison of adolescent suicide victims with suicidal inpatients. Arch Gen Psychiatry 45:581–588, 1988

Brent DA, Perper JA, Allman C, et al: The presence and accessibility of firearms in the homes of adolescent suicides. JAMA 266:2989–2995, 1991

Brent DA, Perper JA, Moritz GM, et al: Firearms and adolescent suicide: a community case-control study. Am J Dis Child 147:1066–1071, 1993

Brodaty H, Andrews G, Austin A: Psychiatric illness in general practice: how is it managed? Aust Fam Physician 11:682–686, 1982

Brown GL, Ebert MH, Goyer PF, et al: Aggression, suicide and serotonin: relationships to CSF amine metabolites. Am J Psychiatry 139:741–746, 1982

Brown HN: Patient suicide during residency training (1): incidence, implications, and program response. Journal of Psychiatric Education 11:201–216, 1987a

Brown HN: The impact of suicide on therapists in training. Compr Psychiatry 28:101–112, 1987b

Brown HN: Patient suicide and therapist training in suicide understanding and responding, in Suicide: Understanding and Responding. Edited by Jacobs D, Brown HN. New York, International Universities Press, 1989

Burdick BM, Holmes CB, Wain RF: Recognition of suicide signs by physicians in different areas of specialization. J Med Educ 58:716–721, 1983

Cantor CH, Lewin T: Firearms and suicide in Australia. Aust N Z J Psychiatry 24:500–509, 1990

Carlson GA, Cantwell DP: Suicidal behavior and depression in children and adolescents. Journal of the American Academy of Child Psychiatry 21:361–368, 1982

Chemtob CM, Bauer GB, Hamada RS, et al: Patient suicide: occupational hazard for psychologists and psychiatrists. Professional Psychology: Research and Practice 20:294–300, 1988a

Chemtob CM, Hamada RS, Bauer G, et al: Patients' suicides: frequency and impact on psychiatrists. Am J Psychiatry 145:224–228, 1988b

Chia BH: Suicide in the young of Singapore. Ann Acad Med Singapore 8:262–268, 1979

Choron J: Suicide. New York, Charles Scribner's Sons, 1972

Clarke RV, Jones PR: Suicide and increased availability of handguns in the United States. Soc Sci Med 28:805–809, 1989

Clarke G, Hawkins W, Murphy M, et al: Prevention of depression in at-risk high school adolescents: a randomized trial of a cognitive therapy intervention. Presentation at the annual meeting of the American Academy of Child and Adolescent Psychiatry, San Antonio, TX, October 1993

Coccaro EF, Siever LJ, Klar HM, et al: Serotonergic studies in patients with affective and personality disorders. Arch Gen Psychiatry 46:587–599, 1989

Cohen P, Kasen S, Brook JS, et al: Diagnostic predictors of treatment patterns in a cohort of adolescents. J Am Acad Child Adolesc Psychiatry 30:989–993, 1991

Coleman L: Suicide Clusters. Boston, MA, Faber & Faber, 1987

Coombs DW, Miller HL, Alarcon R, et al: Communications between parasuicides and caregivers. Suicide Life Threat Behav 22:289–299, 1992

Costello EJ: Primary care pediatrics and child psychopathology: a review of diagnostic, treatment, and referral practices. Pediatrics 78:1044–1051, 1988

Cytryn L, Gershon ES, McKnew DH: Childhood depression: genetic or environmental influences. Integrative Psychiatry 2:17–23, 1984

Davenport JA, Davenport J: Native American suicide: a Durkheimian analysis. Social Casework 68:533–539, 1987

Davidson L, Gould MS: Contagion as a risk factor for youth suicide, in Report of the Secretary's Task Force on Youth Suicide, Vol 2: Risk Factors for Youth Suicide. (DHHS Publ No ADM-89-1622). Washington, DC, U.S. Government Printing Office, 1989

Davidson L, Gould MS: Contagion as a risk factor for youth suicide, in Risk Factors for Youth Suicide. Edited by Davidson L, Linnoila M. New York, Hemisphere, 1991

Davidson S, Ferguson B, Khalis N, et al: Measurement of adolescent suicidal behavior. Presentation at the American Academy of Child and Adolescent Psychiatry, Chicago, IL, October 1990

de Boismont AFB: Du Suicide et de la Folie Suicide. Paris, Librarie Germer Bailliere, 1865

de Catanzano D: Suicide and Self-Damaging Behavior: A Sociobiological Perspective. New York, Academic Press, 1981

Deutsch CJ: Self reported sources of stress among psychotherapists. Professional Psychology: Research and Practice 15:838–845, 1984

DeVos GA: Suicide in cross-cultural perspective, in Suicidal Behavior: Diagnosis and Management. Edited by Resnick HL. Boston, MA, Little, Brown, 1968

de Wilde EJ, Kienhorst ICWM, Diekstra RFW, et al: The relationship between adolescent suicidal behavior and life events in childhood and adolescence. Am J Psychiatry 149:45–51, 1992

Dingman CW, McGlashan TH: Characteristics of patients with serious suicidal intentions who ultimately commit suicide. Hosp Community Psychiatry 39:295–299, 1988

Directory of Graduate Medical Education. Chicago, IL, American Medical Association, 1995–96

Dismang LH, Watson J, May PA: Adolescent suicide at an indian reservation. Am J Orthopsychiatry 44:43–49, 1974

Dryfoos JG: Adolescents at Risk: Prevalence and Prevention. New York, Oxford University Press, 1991

Dudley M, Waters B, Kelk N, et al: Youth suicide in New South Wales: urban–rural trends. Med J Aust 156:83–88, 1992

Durkheim E: Suicide: A Study in Sociology. Glencoe, NY, Free Press, 1951

Dyer JAT, Kreitman N: Hopelessness, depression, and suicidal intent in parasuicide. Br J Psychiatry 144:127–133, 1984

Elster AB, Kuznets NJ: Guidelines for Adolescent Preventive Services. Baltimore, MD, Williams & Wilkins, 1993

Erikson E: Insight and Responsibility. New York, WW Norton, 1964

Erikson EH: Identity, Youth and Crisis. New York, WW Norton, 1968

Esquirol JED: Des Maladies Mentales Consideres sous les Rapports Medicals, Hygeniques et Medico-Legales (1838). English translation by Hunt EK. Mental Maladies: Treatise on Insanity. New York, Hefner, 1965

Farberow NL: Suicide in Different Cultures. Baltimore, MD, University Park Press, 1975

Fingerhut L, Kleinman J: Trends and current status in childhood mortality, U.S. 1900–1985. Vital and Health Statistics. Series 3, No. 26 (DHHS Publ No 89-410). Hyattsville, MD, National Center for Health Statistics, 1989

Fletcher C: Listening and talking to patients: the problem. BMJ 281:845–847, 1980

Forbes LM: Incest, anger, and suicide, in Adolescents Grow in Groups. Edited by Berkovitz IH. New York, Brunner/Mazel, 1972

Friedman RC, Clarkson J, Conn R, et al: DSM III and affective pathology in hospitalized adolescents. J Nerv Ment Dis 170:511–521, 1982

Fyer MR, Frances AJ, Sullivan T, et al: Suicide attempts in patients with borderline personality disorder. Am J Psychiatry 145:737–739, 1988

Gadpaille WJ: Research into the physiology of maleness and femaleness. Arch Gen Psychiatry 26:193–206, 1972

Gadpaille WJ: Cross-species and cross-cultural contributions to the understanding of homosexual activity. Arch Gen Psychiatry 37:349–356, 1980

Gadpaille WJ: Innate masculine/feminine traits: their contributions to conflict. J Am Acad Psychoanal 11:401–424, 1983

Garcia-Preto N: Transformation of the family system in adolescence, in The Changing Family Life Cycle. Edited by Carter B, McGoldrick M. New York, Gardner Press, 1988

Gershon ES, Hamovit JH, Guroff JJ, et al: Birth cohort changes in manic and depressive disorders in relatives of bipolar and schizo-affective patients. Arch Gen Psychiatry 44:314–319, 1987

Gibson P: Gay male and lesbian youth suicide, in Report of the Secretary's Task Force on Youth Suicide, Vol 3, Prevention and Interventions in Youth Suicide (DHHS Publ No ADM-89-1623). Washington, DC, U.S. Government Printing Office, 1989

Gilligan C: In a Different Voice. Cambridge, MA, Harvard University Press, 1982

Gilligan C, Kohlberg L, Lerner J, et al: Moral reasoning about sexual dilemmas, in Technical Report of the Commission on Obscenity and Pornography, Vol 1. Washington, DC, U.S. Government Printing Office, 1971

Gold PW, Goodwin FK, Chrouses GP: Clinical and biochemical manifestations of depression: relation to neurobiology of stress. N Engl J Med 319:348–355, 413–420, 1988

Goldberg D: The recognition of psychiatric illness by non-psychiatrists. Aust N Z J Psychiatry 18:128–134, 1984

Goldstein LS, Buongiorno PA: Psychotherapists as suicide survivors. Am J Psychother 38:392–398, 1984

Gould MS: The role of contagion in adolescent suicide. Rounds presentation at the New York Hospital, Westchester Division, White Plains, NY, March 1992

Gould MS, Shaffer D, Davies M: Truncated pathways from childhood to adulthood: attrition in follow-up studies due to death, in Straight and Devious Pathways from Childhood to Adulthood. Edited by Robins L, Rutter M. Cambridge, England, Cambridge University Press, 1990

Gould MS, Shaffer D, Fishman P, et al: The clinical prediction of adolescent suicide, in Assessment and Prediction of Suicide. Edited by Maris RW, Berman AL, Maltsburger JT, et al. New York, Guilford, 1992

Greenson RR: Disidentifying from mother: its special importance for the boy. Int J Psychoanal 49:370–373, 1968

Grolman EA: Suicide: Prevention, Intervention, and Postvention. Boston, MA, Beacon Press, 1988

Grossman W: Pain, aggression, fantasy, and concepts of sado-masochism. Psychoanal Q 60:22–52, 1991

Group for the Advancement of Psychiatry: Normal Adolescence: Its Dynamics and Impact (GAP Report No 68). New York, Scribner, 1968

Group for the Advancement of Psychiatry: Power and Authority in Adolescence: The Origins and Resolutions of Intergenerational Conflict (GAP Report No 101). New York, Mental Health Materials Center, Inc, 1978

Group for the Advancement of Psychiatry: Crises of Adolescence: Teenage Pregnancy: Impact on Adolescent Development (GAP Report No 118). New York, Brunner/Mazel, 1986

Group for the Advancement of Psychiatry: Suicide and Ethnicity in the United States (GAP Report No 128). New York, Brunner/Mazel, 1989

Grove O, Lynge I: Suicide and attempted suicide in Greenland: a controlled study in Nuuk (Godthaab). Acta Psychiatr Scand 60:375–391, 1979

Gunderson JC: Borderline Personality Disorder. Washington, DC, American Psychiatric Press, 1984

Haggerty RJ: Health policy initiatives in adolescents. Bull N Y Acad Med 67:514–526, 1991

Harkavy-Friedman J, Asnis G, Boeck M, et al: Prevalence of specific suicidal behaviors in a high school sample. Am J Psychiatry 144:1203–1206, 1987

Harry J: Sexual identity issues, in Report of the Secretary's Task Force on Youth Suicide, Vol 2: Risk Factors for Youth Suicide (DHHS Publ No ADM-89-1622). Washington, DC, U.S. Government Printing Office, 1989

Hauser S, Powers S, Noam G, et al: Familial contexts of adolescent ego development. Child Dev 55:195–213, 1984

Hawton K, Blackstock E: General practice aspects of self-poisoning and self-injury. Psychol Med 6:571–575, 1976

Hawton K, Bancroft J, Catalan J, et al: Domiciliary and out-patient treatment of self-poisoning patients by medical and non-medical staff. Psychol Med 11:169–177, 1981

Hawton K, Cole D, O'Grady J, et al: Adolescents who take overdoses: their characteristics, problems, and contacts with helping agencies. Br J Psychiatry 140:118–123, 1982

Hendin H: Suicide: the psychosocial dimension. Suicide Life Threat Behav 8:99–117, 1978

Hendin H: Psychodynamics of suicide, with particular reference to the young. Am J Psychiatry 148:1150–1158, 1991

Henry AF, Short JF: Suicide and Homicide. New York, Free Press, 1954

Henry AF, Short JF: The sociology of suicide, in Clues to Suicide. Edited by Schneidman ES, Farberow NL. New York, McGraw-Hill, 1957

Hickson GB, Altemeier WA, O'Connor S: Concerns of mothers seeking care in private pediatric offices: opportunities for expanding services. Pediatrics 72:619–624, 1983

Hillard JR, Zitek B, Thieuhaus OJ: Residency training in emergency psychiatry: changes between 1980–1990. Academic Psychiatry 17:125–129, 1993

Hippler AE: Fusion and frustration: dimensions in the cross-cultural ethnopsychology of suicide. American Anthropologist 71:1074–1087, 1969

Hoffman L: Foundations of Family Therapy. New York, Basic Books, 1981

Hoffman L: The family life cycle and discontinuous change, in The Changing Family Life Cycle. Edited by Carter B, McGoldrick M. New York, Gardner Press, 1988

Holinger PC, Klemen EH: Violent deaths in the United States, 1900–1975. Soc Sci Med 16:1929–1938, 1982

Holinger PC, Offer D: Prediction of adolescent suicide: a population model. Am J Psychiatry 139:302–307, 1982

Holinger PC, Offer D: Sociodemographic, epidemiologic and individual attributes in alcohol, drug abuse, and mental health administration, in Report of the Secretary's Task Force on Youth Suicide, Vol 2: Risk Factors for Youth Suicide (DHHS Publ No ADM-89-1622). Washington, DC, U.S. Government Printing Office, 1989

Huffine C: Social and cultural risk factors for youth suicide, in Report of the Secretary's Task Force on Youth Suicide, Vol 2: Risk Factors for Youth Suicide (DHHS Publ No ADM-89-1622). Washington, DC, U.S. Government Printing Office, 1989

Inhelder B, Piaget J: The Growth of Logical Thinking from Childhood to Adolescence. New York, Basic Books, 1958

Inman DA, Bascue LO, Kahn WJ: The relationship between suicide knowledge and suicide intervention skill. Death Educ 8:179–184, 1984

Jacobsen AM, Goldberg ID, Burns BJ, et al: Diagnosed mental disorder in children and use of health services in four organized health care settings. Am J Psychiatry 137:559–565, 1980

Jeffries MDW: Samsonic suicide or suicide of revenge among Africans. African Studies 11:118–122, 1952

Jilek-Aall L: Suicidal behavior among youth: a cross-cultural comparison. Transcultural Psychiatric Research Review 25:87–105, 1988

Johnson RL, Sheir DK: Sexual victimization of boys: experience at an adolescent medicine clinic. J Adolesc Health 6:372–376, 1985

Joint Commission on Mental Health of Children: Crisis in Child Mental Health: Challenge for the 1970's. New York, Harper & Row, 1969

Jones EF, Forrest JD, Goldman N, et al: Teenage pregnancy in developed countries: determinants and policy implications. Fam Plann Perspect 17:53–63, 1985

Jones FA Jr: Therapists as survivors of client suicide, in Suicide and Its Aftermath. Edited by Dunne JD, McIntosh JL, Dunne-Maxim K. New York, WW Norton, 1987

Jones JS, Stanley B, Mann J, et al: CSF 5 HIAA and HVA concentrations in elderly depressed patients who attempted suicide. Am J Psychiatry 147:1225–1227, 1990

Juel-Nielsen N, Videbach T: A twin study of suicide. Acta Genet Med Gemellol (Roma) 19:307–310, 1970

Kahn MW: Cultural clash and psychopathology in three aboriginal cultures. Academic Psychology Bulletin 4:553–561, 1982

Kahne MJ: Suicide among patients in mental hospitals: a study of the psychiatrists who conducted their psychotherapy. Psychiatry 31:32–43, 1968

Kalafat J, Elias M: Adolescents' experience with and response to suicidal teens. Suicide Life Threat Behav 22:314–321, 1992

Kallmann F, Anastasio M: Twin studies on the psychopathology of suicide. J Nerv Ment Dis 105:40–55, 1947

Kaplan HI, Sadock BJ: Suicide. Synopsis of Psychiatry, 6th Edition. Baltimore, MD, Williams & Wilkins, 1991

Kasdin AE, French MR, Uris AS, et al: Hopelessness, depression, and suicidal intent among psychiatrically disturbed inpatient children. J Consult Clin Psychol 51:504–510, 1983

Kellerman AL, Rivara FP, Somes G, et al: Suicide in the home in relationship to gun ownership. N Engl J Med 327:467–472, 1992

Kernberg OF: Suicidal behavior in borderline patients: diagnosis and psychotherapeutic considerations. Presented at the Symposium on Suicide and the Borderline Patient, American Psychiatric Association Annual Meeting, New Orleans, LA, May 1991

Kernberg P: The analysis of a fifteen and a half year old girl with suicidal tendencies, in The Analyst and the Adolescent at Work. Edited by Harley M. New York, New York Times Book Company, 1974

Killias M: International correlations between gun ownership and rates of homicide and suicide. Can Med Assoc J 148:1721–1725, 1993

Kim WJ: Psychiatric aspects of epileptic children and adolescents. J Am Acad Child Adolesc Psychiatry 30:874–886, 1991

Kitamura A: Suicide and attempted suicide among children and adolescents. Pediatrician 12:73–79, 1983–85

Kohlberg L, Gilligan C: The adolescent as a philosopher: the discovery of the self in a postconventional world. Daedalus 100:1051–1086, 1971

Kraepelin E: Dementia Praecox and Schizophrenia (1913). Translated by Barclay RM. Huntington, NY, R. E. Krieger Publishing, 1971

Kruesi MJP: Cruelty to animals and CSF 5-HIAA. Psychiatry Res 28:115–116, 1989

Kruesi MJP, Rapoport JL, Hamburger S, et al: CSF monoamine metabolites, aggression and impulsivity in disruptive behavior disorders of children and adolescents. Arch Gen Psychiatry 47:419–426, 1990

Landau J: Therapy with families in cultural transition, in Ethnicity and Family Therapy. Edited by McGoldrick M, Pearce JK, Giordano J. New York, Guilford, 1982

Landau-Stanton J, Stanton MD: Treating suicidal adolescents and their families, in Handbook of Adolescents and Family Therapy. Edited by Mirkin MP, Koman SL. New York, Gardner Press, 1985

Lester D: Gun ownership and suicide in the United States. Psychol Med 19:519–521, 1989

Lester D: The availability of firearms and the use of firearms for suicide: a study of 20 countries. Acta Psychiatr Scand 81:146–147, 1990

Lester D, Murrel MD: The preventive effect of strict gun control laws on suicide and homicide. Suicide Life Threat Behav 12:131–140, 1982

Li WL: A comparative study of suicide. International Journal of Comparative Sociology 12:281–286, 1971

Linehan NN: Suicidal people: one population or two? Psychobiology of suicidal behavior. Ann N Y Acad Sci 487:16–33, 1986

Litman RE: When patients commit suicide. Am J Psychother 19:570–576, 1965

Loftin C, McDowall D, Wiersema B, et al: Effects of restrictive licensing of handguns on homicide and suicide in the District of Columbia. N Engl J Med 325:1615–1620, 1991

Lomax WJ: A proposed curriculum on suicide care for psychiatry residency. Suicide Life Threat Behav 16:56–64, 1986

Long KA: Suicide intervention and prevention with indian adolescent populations. Issues Ment Health Nurs 8:247–253, 1986

Maltsberger JT: The implications of patient suicide for the surviving psychotherapist, in Suicide and Clinical Practice. Edited by Jacobs D. Washington, DC, American Psychiatric Press, 1992, pp 169–182

Maris RW: Suicide intervention: the existential and biomedical perspectives, in Suicide: Understanding and Responding. Edited by Jacobs D, Brown HN. Madison, CT, International Universities Press, 1989

Marohn R: Adolescent rebellion and the task of separation. Adolesc Psychiatry 8:173–183, 1980

Marzuk PM, Tierney H, Tardiff K, et al: Increased risk of suicide in persons with AIDS. JAMA 259:1333–1337, 1988

Masamura WT: Social integration and suicide: a test of Durkheim's theory. Behavioral Science Research 12:251–269, 1977

McElroy SL, Hudson JI, Pope HG, et al: The DSM-III-R impulse control disorders not elsewhere classified: clinical characteristics and relationship to other psychiatric disorders. Am J Psychiatry 149:318–327, 1992

McGoldrick M, Walsh F: A systemic view of family history and loss, in Group and Family Therapy. Edited by Aronson M. New York, Brunner/Mazel, 1983

McGuinies E, Nordholm LA, Ward CD, et al: Sex and cultural differences in perceived locus of control among students in five countries. J Consult Clin Psychol 42:451–455, 1974

Meltzer HY, Lowy MT: The serotonin hypothesis of depression, in Psychopharmacology: Third Generation of Progress. Edited by Meltzer HY. New York, Ruben Press, 1987

Miller SI, Shoenfield LS: Suicide attempt patterns among the Navajo indians. Int J Soc Psychiatry 17:189–193, 1971

Miller S, Rotheram-Borus MJ, Piacentini J, et al: Successful Negotiation Acting Positively. New York, Columbia University Press, 1992

Mufson L, Moreau D, Weissman M, et al: Interpersonal Therapy for Depressed Adolescents. New York, Guilford, 1993

Murphy GE, Wetzel RD: Suicide risk by birth cohort in the United States, 1949–1974. Arch Gen Psychiatry 37:519–523, 1980

Murphy GE, Armstrong JW, Hermele SL, et al: Suicide and alcoholism: interpersonal loss confirmed as a predictor. Arch Gen Psychiatry 36:65–69, 1979

National Academy of Sciences, Institute of Medicine, Division of Mental Health and Behavioral Medicine: Research on Children's and Adolescents' Mental, Behavioral and Developmental Disorders: Mobilizing a National Initiative. Washington, DC, National Academy Press, 1989

National Center for Health Statistics, Department of Health and Human Services, Mortality Statistics Branch: Vital Statistics of the United States, 1960, Vol 2, Part B. Washington, DC, U.S. Government Printing Office, 1963

National Center for Health Statistics, Department of Health and Human Services, Mortality Statistics Branch: Vital Statistics of the United States, 1970, Vol 2, Part B. Washington, DC, U.S. Government Printing Office, 1974

National Center for Health Statistics, Department of Health and Human Services, Mortality Statistics Branch: Vital Statistics of the United States, 1980, Vol 2, Part B. Washington, DC, U.S. Government Printing Office, 1985

National Center for Health Statistics, Department of Health and Human Services, Mortality Statistics Branch: Vital Statistics of the United States, 1990, Vol 2, Part B. Washington, DC, U.S. Government Printing Office, 1994

Neuringer D: Rigid thinking in suicidal individuals. J Consult Psychol 28:54–58, 1964

Norton EM, Durlak JA, Richards MH: Peer knowledge of and reactions to adolescent suicide. Journal of Youth and Adolescence 18:427–437, 1989

Nurcome B: Malpractice, in Child and Adolescent Psychiatry: A Comprehensive Textbook. Edited by Lewis M. Baltimore, MD, Williams & Wilkins, 1991

Offord DR, Boyle MH, Szatmari P, et al: Ontario child health study, II: six-month prevalence of disorder and rates of service utilization. Arch Gen Psychiatry 44:832–836, 1987

Orbach I, Feshbach S, Carlson G, et al: Attraction and repulsion by life and death in suicidal and in normal children. J Consult Clin Psychol 51:661–670, 1983

Orbach I, Rosenham E, Harry E: Some aspects of cognitive functioning in suicidal children. J Am Acad Child Adolesc Psychiatry 26:181–185, 1987

Ortega y Gasset J: The Revolt of the Masses. New York, WW Norton, 1932

Pallis DJ, Barraclough BM, Levey AB, et al: Estimating suicide risk among attempted suicides: the development of new clinical scales. Br J Psychiatry 141:37–44, 1982

Patsiokas A, Clum G, Luscomb R: Cognitive characteristics in suicide attempters. J Consult Clin Psychol 47:478–484, 1979

Paul NL, Grosser GH: Operational mourning and its role in conjoint marital therapy. Community Ment Health J 1:345–389, 1965

Paykel ES: Stress and life events, in Report of the Secretary's Task Force on Youth Suicide, Vol 2: Risk Factors for Youth Suicide (DHHS Publ No ADM-89-1622). Washington, DC, U.S. Government Printing Office, 1989

Peck ML: Youth suicide: programs for prevention, intervention, and postvention, in Expanding Mental Health Interventions in Schools. Edited by Berkovitz IH, Seliger JS. Dubuque, IO, Kendall/Hunt, 1985

Perrin J, Guyer B, Lawrence JM: Health care services for children and adolescents. The Future of Children, 2. Los Altos, CA, Center for the Future of Children, The David and Lucille Packard Foundation, 1992

Peterson LG, Bongar G: Training physicians in the clinical evaluation of the suicidal patient, in Methods in Teaching Consultation-Liaison Psychiatry, Vol 20: Advances in Psychosomatic Medicine. Edited by Hale MS. Basel, Karger, 1990

Pfeffer CP, Zuckerman S, Plutchik R, et al: Suicidal behaviors in normal school children: a comparison with child psychiatric inpatients. J Am Acad Child Adolesc Psychiatry 23:416–423, 1984

Pfeffer CP, Newcorn I, Kaplan G, et al: Suicidal behavior in adolescent psychiatric inpatients. J Am Acad Child Adolesc Psychiatry 27:357–361, 1988

Plutchik R, van Praag HM: Psychosocial correlates of suicide and violence risk, in Violence and Suicidality. Edited by van Praag HM, Plutchik R, Apter A. New York, Brunner/Mazel, 1990

Puig-Antich J, Goetz R, Hanlon C, et al: Sleep architecture and REM sleep measures in prepubertal major depressives. Arch Gen Psychiatry 36:187–192, 1983

Pynoos RS, Eth S: Children traumatized by witnessing acts of violence: homicide, rape, or suicide behavior, in Post-Traumatic Stress Disorder in Children. Edited by Eth S, Pynoos RS. Washington, DC, American Psychiatric Press, 1985, pp 17–43

Resnick HLP: Psychological resynthesis: a clinical approach to the survivors of a death by suicide, in Aspects of Depression. Edited by Schneidman ES, Ortega M. Boston, MA, Little, Brown, 1969

Rich AR, Bonner RL: Concurrent validity of a stress-vulnerability model of suicidal ideation and behavior: a follow-up study. Suicide Life Threat Behav 17:265–270, 1987

Rich CL, Young D, Fowler RC: San Diego suicide study, I: young vs. old cases. Arch Gen Psychiatry 43:577–582, 1986

Rich CL, Fowler RC, Fogarty LA, et al: San Diego suicide study: relationships between diagnoses and stressors. Arch Gen Psychiatry 45:589–592, 1988

Rich CL, Young JG, Fowler RC, et al: Guns and suicide: possible effects of some specific legislation. Am J Psychiatry 147:342–346, 1990

Robins E, Murphy GE, Wilkinson RH Jr, et al: Some clinical considerations in the prevention of suicide based on a study of 134 successful suicides. Am J Public Health 49:888–899, 1959

Rockwell DA, O'Brien W: Physicians' knowledge and attitudes about suicide. JAMA 225:1347–1349, 1973

Rosen DH: The serious suicide attempt: five year follow-up study of 886 patients. JAMA 235:2105–2109, 1976

Rosenberg M, Smith J, Davidson L, et al: The emergence of youth suicide: an epidemiologic analysis and public health perspective. Ann Rev Public Health 8:417–427, 1987

Rotheram-Borus MJ, Trautman PD: Hopelessness, depression, and suicidal intent among adolescent suicide attempters. J Am Acad Child Adolesc Psychiatry 27:700–704, 1988

Roy A: Family history of suicide. Arch Gen Psychiatry 40:971–974, 1983

Roy A: Suicide, in Comprehensive Textbook of Psychiatry, 5th Edition. Edited by Kaplan HI, Sadock BJ. Baltimore, MD, Williams & Wilkins, 1989

Roy A: Genetics and suicidal behavior, in Risk Factors for Youth Suicide. Edited by Davidson L, Linnoila M. New York, Hemisphere, 1991

Rubinstein DH: A stress-diathesis theory of suicide. Suicide Life Threat Behav 16:182–197, 1986

Rubinstein JL, Heeren T, Houseman D, et al: Suicidal behavior in "normal" adolescents: risks and protective factors. Am J Orthopsychiatry 59:59–71, 1989

Sathyavathi K: Suicide among children in Bangalore. Indian J Pediatr 42:149–157, 1975

Schneidman E: An overview: personality, motivation, and behavior theories, in Suicide Theory and Clinical Aspects. Edited by Hankoff LD. Littleton, MA, PSG Publishing, 1979

Schulsinger F, Kety SS, Rosenthal D, et al: A family study of suicide, in Origin, Prevention, and Treatment of Affective Disorders. Edited by Schou M, Stromgren E. New York, Academic Press, 1979

Shaffer D: Suicide in childhood and early adolescence. J Child Psychol Psychiatry 15:275–291, 1974

Shaffer D: Depression, mania, and suicidal acts, in Child Psychiatry: Modern Approaches, 2nd Edition. Edited by Rutter M, Herson L. Oxford, Blackwell Press, 1985

Shaffer D: Suicide: risk factors and the public health. Am J Public Health 83:171–172, 1993

Shaffer D, Fisher P: The epidemiology of suicide in children and young adolescents. Journal of the American Academy of Child Psychiatry 20:545–565, 1981

Shaffer D, Gould M: Study of Completed and Attempted Suicides in Adolescents. Progress Report. Washington, DC, National Institute of Mental Health, 1987

Shaffer D, Hicks R: Suicide and attempted suicide in adolescents, in The Textbook of Adolescent Medicine. Edited by McAnerney E, Orr DP, Kreipe RE, et al. Philadelphia, PA, WB Saunders, 1992

Shaffer D, Garland NA, Gould M, et al: Preventing teenage suicide: a critical review. J Am Acad Child Adolesc Psychiatry 27:675–687, 1988

Shaffer D, Gould MS, Fisher P: Psychiatric diagnosis in child and adolescent suicide. Arch Gen Psychiatry (in press)

Shafii M: Completed suicide in children and adolescents: methods of psychological autopsy, in Suicide Among Youth. Edited by Pfeffer CR. Washington, DC, American Psychiatric Press, 1989, pp 1–19

Shapiro ER, Freedman J: Family dynamics of adolescent suicide, in Adolescent Psychiatry, Vol 14. Edited by Feinstein S. Chicago, IL, University of Chicago Press, 1987

Shein HM: Suicide care: obstacles in the education of psychiatry residents. Omega 7:75–81, 1976

Shore JH: American indian suicide—fact and fantasy. Psychiatry 38:86–91, 1975

Shuppert SM: Office Visits to Psychiatrists: United States, 1989–90; Advance Data from Vital and Health Statistics (Report No 237). Hyattsville, MD, National Center for Health Statistics, 1993

Sloan JH, Rivara FP, Reay DT, et al: Firearms regulation and the rates of suicide: a comparison of two metropolitan areas. N Engl J Med 322:369–373, 1990

Smilkstein G: The family APGAR: a proposal for a family function test and its use by physicians. J Fam Pract 6:1231–1239, 1978

Smith DH, Hackathorn L: Some social and psychological factors related to suicide in primitive societies: a cross-cultural comparative study. Suicide Life Threat Behav 12:195–211, 1982

Smith K, Crawford S: Suicidal behavior among "normal" high school students. Suicide Life Threat Behav 16:313–325, 1986

Solomon MI, Hellon CP: Suicide and age in Alberta, Canada. Arch Gen Psychiatry 37:511–513, 1980

Sorensen T, Snow B: How children tell: the process of disclosure in child sexual abuse. Child Welfare 70:3–15, 1991

Stack S: Suicide, a comparative analysis. Social Forces 57:644–653, 1978

Stanley M, Mann JJ: Biological factors associated with suicide, in American Psychiatric Press Review of Psychiatry, Vol 7. Edited by Frances AJ, Hales RE. Washington, DC, American Psychiatric Press, 1988, pp 334–352

Starfield B, Borkowf S: Physicians' recognition of complaints made by parents about their children's health. Pediatrics 43:168–172, 1969

Stein B, Golombek H, Morton P, et al: Personality functioning and change in clinical presentation from early to late adolescence. Adolesc Psychiatry 14:378–393, 1987

Sterlin H: Separating Parents and Adolescents: A Perspective on Running Away, Schizophrenia, and Waywardness. New York, Quadrangle Press, 1974

Stern DN: Interpersonal World of the Infant. New York, Basic Books, 1985

Stevenson K, Maholick M: Child and Adolescent Psychiatry: Guidelines for Treatment Resources, Quality Assurance, Peer Review and Reimbursement. Washington, DC, American Academy of Child and Adolescent Psychiatry, 1987

Stiffman AR, Felton E, Robins LN, et al: Problems and health-seeking in high-risk adolescent patients of health clinics. J Adolesc Health Care 9:305–309, 1988

Stoller RJ: Symbiosis anxiety and the development of masculinity. Arch Gen Psychiatry 30:164–172, 1974

Stone MH: The P.I. 500. New York, Guilford, 1989

Stone MH: The Fate of Borderline Patients. New York, Guilford, 1990

Stone MH: Suicide in borderline and other adolescents. Adolesc Psychiatry 18:289–305, 1992

Sudak HS, Ford AB, Rushforth NB: Adolescent suicide: an overview. Am J Psychother 38:350–363, 1984

Sugar M: Psychotherapy with the adolescent in self-selected peer groups, in Adolescents Grow in Groups. Edited by Berkovitz IH. New York, Brunner/Mazel, 1972

Tischler CL, McKenry PC, Morgan KC: Adolescent suicide attempts: some significant factors. Suicide Life Threat Behav 11:86–92, 1981

Tsuang MT: Suicide in schizophrenics, manics, depressives, and surgical controls: a comparison with general population suicide mortality. Arch Gen Psychiatry 35:153–155, 1978

Tsuang MT: Risk of suicide in the relatives of schizophrenics, manics, depressives, and controls. J Clin Psychiatry 44:396–400, 1983

U.S. Congress, Office of Technology Assessment: Adolescent Health, Vol I: Summary and Policy Options, and Vol II: Background and the Effectiveness of Selected Prevention and Treatment Services (OTA-H-466). Washington, DC, U.S. Government Printing Office, 1991

U.S. Department of Health and Human Services; Public Health Service; Alcohol, Drug Abuse, and Mental Health Administration; National Institute of Mental Health: Report of the Secretary's Task Force on Youth Suicide, Vol I: Overview and Recommendations. Washington, DC, U.S. Government Printing Office, 1989a

U.S. Department of Health and Human Services; Public Health Service; Alcohol, Drug Abuse, and Mental Health Administration; National Institute of Mental Health: Report of the Secretary's Task Force on Youth Suicide, Vol 2: Risk Factors for Youth Suicide (DHHS Publ No ADM-89-1622). Washington, DC, U.S. Government Printing Office, 1989b

Van Praag HM, Plutchik R, Conte H: The serotonin hypothesis of (auto) aggression: critical appraisal of the evidence. Ann N Y Acad Sci 487:150–157, 1986

Van Winkle NW, May PA: Native American suicide in New Mexico, 1957–1979; a comparative study. Hum Organ 45:296–309, 1986

Vigderhous G, Fishman G: Socioeconomic determinants of female suicide rates: a cross-national comparison. International Review of Modern Sociology 7:199–211, 1977

Virkkunen M, Nuutila A, Goodwin FK, et al: Cerebrospinal fluid monoamine metabolite levels in male arsonists. Arch Gen Psychiatry 44:241–247, 1987

Vital Statistics of the United States, 1979: Mortality. Washington, DC, U.S. Government Printing Office, 1984

von Goethe JW: The Sorrows of Young Werther and Novella. Translated by Mayer E, Bogan L. New York, Vintage Books, 1990

Walsh F, Scheinkman M: The family context of adolescence, in Handbook of Clinical Research and Practice with Adolescents. Edited by Tolan PH, Cohler BJ. New York, Wiley-Interscience, 1993

Ward JA, Fox JA: A suicide epidemic on an indian reserve. Can J Psychiatry 22:423–426, 1977

Weissberg M: The meagerness of physicians' training in emergency psychiatric intervention. Acad Med 65:747–750, 1990

Weissman M: The epidemiology of suicide attempts, 1960 to 1971. Arch Gen Psychiatry 30:737–746, 1974

Weissman M, Fox K, Klerman GL: Hostility and depression associated with suicide attempts. Am J Psychiatry 130:450–455, 1973

Whitaker A, Shaffer D: Suicidal ideation in a non-referred adolescent population. Presented at the Roddy Brickell Symposium at the New York State Psychiatric Institute, March 16, 1993

Whitaker A, Johnson J, Shaffer D, et al: Uncommon troubles in young people: prevalence estimates of selected psychiatric disorders in a non-referred adolescent population. Arch Gen Psychiatry 47:487–496, 1990

GAP Committees and Membership

Committee on Adolescence

Richard C. Marohn, Chicago, IL, *Chairperson*
Ian A. Canino, New York, NY
Warren J. Gadpaille, Denver, CO
Harvey Horowitz, Philadelphia, PA
Sarah Huertas-Goldman, San Juan, PR
Paulina F. Kernberg, New York, NY
Clarice J. Kestenbaum, New York, NY
Silvio J. Onesti, Jr., Belmont, MA

Committee on Aging

Gene D. Cohen, Washington, DC, *Chairperson*
Karen Blank, West Hartford, CT
Charles M. Gaitz, Houston, TX
Gary Gottlieb, Philadelphia, PA
Ira R. Katz, Philadelphia, PA
Andrew F. Leuchter, Los Angeles, CA
Gabe J. Maletta, Minneapolis, MN
Richard A. Margolin, Nashville, TN
Kenneth M. Sakauye, New Orleans, LA
Charles A. Shamoian, Larchmont, NY
F. Conyers Thompson, Jr., Atlanta, GA

Committee on Cultural Psychiatry

Ezra Griffith, New Haven, CT, *Chairperson*
Edward Foulks, New Orleans, LA
Francis Lu, San Francisco, CA
Pedro Ruiz, Houston, TX
Ronald Wintrob, Providence, RI
Joe Yamamoto, Los Angeles, CA

Committee on Disabilities

Meyer S. Gunther, Chicago, IL, *Chairperson*
Bryan King, Los Angeles, CA
Robert S. Nesheim, Duluth, MN
William H. Sack, Portland, OR
William A. Sonis, Philadelphia, PA
Margaret L. Stuber, Los Angeles, CA
Henry H. Work, Bethesda, MD

Committee on the Family

Frederick Gottlieb, Los Angeles, CA, *Chairperson*
W. Robert Beavers, Dallas, TX
Henry U. Grunebaum, Cambridge, MA
Herta A. Guttman, Montreal, PQ
Judith Landau-Stanton, Rochester, NY
Ann L. Price, Avon, CT

Committee on Government Policy

Roger Peele, Washington, DC, *Chairperson*
Thomas L. Clannon, San Francisco, CA
Naomi Heller, Washington, DC
John P. D. Shemo, Charlottesville, VA
William W. Van Stone, Washington, DC
Alan Zientes, Washington, DC

Committee on Human Sexuality

Bertram H. Schaffner, New York, NY, *Chairperson*
Paul L. Adams, Louisville, KY

Steven S. Sharfstein, Baltimore, MD
Altha Stewart, New York, NY
Michael Vergare, Philadelphia, PA
George F. Wilson, Somerville, NJ
Jack A. Wolford, Pittsburgh, PA

Committee on Occupational Psychiatry

David B. Robbins, Chappaqua, NY, *Chairperson*
Peter L. Brill, Radnor, PA
Barrie S. Greiff, Newton, MA
Duane Q. Hagen, St. Louis, MO
R. Edward Huffman, Asheville, NC
Robert Larsen, San Francisco, CA
David E. Morrison, Palatine, IL
Jay B. Rohrlich, New York, NY
Clarence J. Rowe, St. Paul, MN
Jeffrey L. Speller, Cambridge, MA

Committee on Planning and Communications

Robert W. Gibson, Towson, MD, *Chairperson*
C. Knight Aldrich, Charlottesville, VA
Allan Beigel, Tucson, AZ
Doyle I. Carson, Dallas, TX
Paul J. Fink, Philadelphia, PA
Robert S. Garber, Longboat Key, FL
Harvey L. Ruben, New Haven, CT
Melvin Sabshin, Washington, DC
Michael R. Zales, Tucson, AZ

Committee on Preventive Psychiatry

Naomi Rae-Grant, London, ON, *Chairperson*
Viola W. Bernard, New York, NY
Stephen Fleck, New Haven, CT
Brian J. McConville, Cincinnati, OH
David R. Offord, Hamilton, ON
Morton M. Silverman, Chicago, IL
Warren T. Vaughan, Jr., Portola Valley, CA

Robert A. Dorwart, Cambridge, MA
James M. Ellison, Watertown, MA
Howard H. Goldman, Potomac, MD
Samuel G. Siris, Glen Oaks, NY

Committee on Public Education

Steven E. Katz, New York, NY, *Chairperson*
David Baron, Ambler, PA
Jack W. Bonner III, Asheville, NC
Jeffrey L. Geller, Worcester, MA
Jeanne Leventhal, Hayward, CA
David Preven, New York, NY
Elise K. Richman, Scarsdale, NY
Boris G. Rifkin, Branford, CT
Andrew E. Slaby, Summit, NJ
Robert A. Solow, Los Angeles, CA
Calvin R. Sumner, Buckhannon, WV
Laurence Tancredi, New York, NY

Committee on Research

Zebulon Taintor, New York, NY, *Chairperson*
Robert Cancro, New York, NY
Russell Gardner, Galveston, TX
John H. Greist, Madison, WI
Jerry M. Lewis, Dallas, TX
John G. Looney, Durham, NC

Committee on Social Issues

Martha J. Kirkpatrick, Los Angeles, CA, *Chairperson*
Ian E. Alger, New York, NY
William R. Beardslee, Waban, MA
Roderic Gorney, Los Angeles, CA
H. James Lurie, Seattle, WA
Ted Nadelson, Boston, MA
Perry Ottenberg, Philadelphia, PA
Kendon W. Smith, Pearl River, NY

Committee on Therapeutic Care

Alan Gruenberg, Philadelphia, PA, *Chairperson*
Bernard Bandler, Cambridge, MA
Thomas E. Curtis, Chapel Hill, NC
Donald C. Fidler, Morgantown, WV
Donald W. Hammersley, Washington, DC
William B. Hunter III, Albuquerque, NM
Milton Kramer, Cincinnati, OH
John Lipkin, Perry Point, MA
William W. Richards, Anchorage, AK

Committee on Therapy

Susan Lazar, Washington, DC, *Chairperson*
Gerald Adler, Boston, MA
Jules R. Bemporad, White Plains, NY
Eugene B. Feigelson, Brooklyn, NY
Andrew P. Morrison, Cambridge, MA
William C. Offenkrantz, Scottsdale, AZ
Allan D. Rosenblatt, La Jolla, CA
Robert Waldinger, West Newton, MA

GINSBURG FELLOWS

Arlener Artis-Trower, Silver Spring, MD *(Committee on Therapeutic Care)*
Elizabeth C. Druss, Cambridge, MA *(Committee on Psychopathology)*
Louis Michel Elie, LaSalle, Quebec, Canada *(Committee on Aging)*
Ryan Finkenbine, Charleston, SC *(Committee on Social Issues)*
Risa Fishman, New York, NY *(Committee on Alcoholism and the Addictions)*
Anna Lucy Fitzgerald, Brighton, MA *(Committee on Cultural Psychiatry)*
Michael Golding, Carrboro, NC *(Committee on Government Policy)*
Scott A. Haas, Louisville, KY *(Committee on Psychiatry and the Law)*
Jacqueline Haimes, Silver Spring, MD *(Committee on Planning and Communications)*
Samia Hasan, Baltimore, MD *(Committee on College Students)*
Lyudmila Karlin, Great Neck, NY *(Committee on Psychiatry and the Community)*
Vassilis Koliatsos, Baltimore, MD *(Committee on Research)*
Heather Krell, Philadelphia, PA *(Committee on Disabilities)*
Patricia Lester, San Francisco, CA *(Committee on Adolescence)*

Mercedes Martinez, Chicago, IL *(Committee on Child Psychiatry)*
Michael Fuller McBride, Milwaukee, WI *(Committee on Public Education)*
Alan Newman, Little Rock, AR *(Committee on International Relations)*
Robert Rogan, Greenville, NC *(Committee on Occupational Psychiatry)*
Jennifer Felice Schreiber, New York, NY *(Committee on Medical Education)*
Roseanne State, Pacific Palisades, CA *(Committee on Therapy)*
Teresa M. Stathas, Columbia, SC *(Committee on Psychiatry and Religion)*
Lynelle Thomas, New Haven, CT *(Committee on Preventive Psychiatry)*
Anna Viltz, Houston, TX *(Committee on Human Sexuality)*
Kenneth William Wilson, New York, NY *(Committee on Mental Health Services)*
Larry Wissow, Baltimore, MD *(Committee on the Family)*

CONTRIBUTING MEMBERS

Gene Abroms, Ardmore, PA
Carlos C. Alden, Jr., Buffalo, NY
Kenneth Z. Altshuler, Dallas, TX
Francis F. Barnes, Washington, DC
Spencer Bayles, Houston, TX
C. Christian Beels, New York, NY
Elissa P. Benedek, Ann Arbor, MI
Renee L. Binder, San Francisco, CA
Mark Blotcky, Dallas, TX
H. Keith H. Brodie, Durham, NC
Charles M. Bryant, San Francisco, CA
Ewald W. Busse, Durham, NC
Robert N. Butler, New York, NY
Eugene M. Caffey, Jr., Bowie, MD
Robert J. Campbell, New York, NY
James P. Cattell, San Diego, CA
Ian L. W. Clancey, Maitland, ON
Sanford I. Cohen, Coral Gables, FL
Lee Combrinck-Graham, Evanston, IL
Robert E. Drake, Hanover, NH
James S. Eaton, Jr., Washington, DC
Lloyd C. Elam, Nashville, TN
Joseph T. English, New York, NY
Sherman C. Feinstein, Highland Park, IL
Archie R. Foley, New York, NY
Henry J. Gault, Highland Park, IL

Richard K. Goodstein, Belle Mead, NJ
*Alexander Gralnick, Port Chester, NY
Milton Greenblatt, Sylmar, CA
Lawrence F. Greenleigh, Los Angeles, CA
Stanley I. Greenspan, Bethesda, MD
Jon E. Gudeman, Milwaukee, WI
William Hetznecker, Merion Station, PA
Johanna A. Hoffman, Scottsdale, AZ
Edward J. Khantzian, Haverhill, MA
James A. Knight, New Orleans, LA
Othilda M. Krug, Cincinnati, OH
Anthony F. Lehman, Baltimore, MD
Alan I. Levenson, Tucson, AZ
Norman L. Loux, Sellersville, PA
Albert J. Lubin, Woodside, CA
John Mack, Chestnut Hill, MA
John A. MacLeod, Cincinnati, OH
Charles A. Malone, Barrington, RI
Peter A. Martin, Lake Orion, MI
Alan A. McLean, Gig Harbor, WA
David Mendell, Houston, TX
Mary E. Mercer, Nyack, NY
Derek Miller, Chicago, IL
Steven M. Mirin, Belmont, MA
Richard D. Morrill, Boston, MA
Robert J. Nathan, Philadelphia, PA
Joseph D. Noshpitz, Washington, DC
Mortimer Ostow, Bronx, NY
Bernard L. Pacella, New York, NY
Herbert Pardes, New York, NY
Norman L. Paul, Lexington, MA
Marvin E. Perkins, Salem, VA
George H. Pollock, Chicago, IL
Becky Potter, Tucson, AZ
David N. Ratnavale, Bethesda, MD
*W. Donald Ross, Cincinnati, OH
Loren Roth, Pittsburgh, PA
Charles Shagass, Philadelphia, PA

---

*Deceased.

Albert J. Silverman, Ann Arbor, MI
Benson R. Snyder, Cambridge, MA
David A. Soskis, Bala Cynwyd, PA
Jeffrey L. Speller, Cambridge, MA
Jeanne Spurlock, Washington, DC
Brandt F. Steele, Denver, CO
Alan A. Stone, Cambridge, MA
Perry C. Talkington, Dallas, TX
John A. Talbott, Baltimore, MD
Bryce Templeton, Philadelphia, PA
Prescott W. Thompson, Portland, OR
John A. Turner, San Francisco, CA
Andrew S. Watson, Ann Arbor, MI
Paul Tyler Wilson, Bethesda, MD
Ann Marie Wolf-Schatz, Conshohocken, PA
Kent A. Zimmerman, Menlo Park, CA
Howard Zonana, New Haven, CT

LIFE MEMBERS

C. Knight Aldrich, Charlottesville, VA
Robert L. Arnstein, Hamden, CT
Bernard Bandler, Cambridge, MA
Walter E. Barton, Hartland, VT
Viola W. Bernard, New York, NY
Henry W. Brosin, Tucson, AZ
John Donnelly, Hartford, CT
Merrill T. Eaton, Omaha, NE
O. Spurgeon English, Narberth, PA
Stephen Fleck, New Haven, CT
Jerome Frank, Baltimore, MD
Robert S. Garber, Longboat Key, FL
Robert I. Gibson, Towson, MD
Margaret M. Lawrence, Pomona, NY
Jerry M. Lewis, Dallas, TX
Harold I. Lief, Philadelphia, PA
Judd Marmor, Los Angeles, CA
Herbert C. Modlin, Topeka, KS
John C. Nemiah, Hanover, NH
William C. Offenkrantz, Scottsdale, AZ

Past Presidents
    *William C. Menninger   1946–51
    Jack R. Ewalt   1951–53
    Walter E. Barton   1953–55
    *Sol W. Ginsburg   1955–57
    *Dana L. Farnsworth   1957–59
    *Marion E. Kenworthy   1959–61
    Henry W. Brosin   1961–63
    *Leo H. Bartemeier   1963–65
    Robert S. Garber   1965–67
    Herbert C. Modlin   1967–69
    John Donnelly   1969–71
    George Tarjan   1971–73
    Judd Marmor   1973–75
    John C. Nemiah   1975–77
    Jack A. Wolford   1977–79
    Robert W. Gibson   1979–81
    *Jack Weinberg   1981–82
    Henry H. Work   1982–85
    Michael R. Zales   1985–87
    Jerry M. Lewis   1987–89
    Carolyn B. Robinowitz   1989–91
    Allan Beigel   1991–93
    John Schowalter   1993–1995

PUBLICATIONS BOARD

Chairperson
    Allan Beigel
    P.O. Box 43460
    Tucson, AZ   85733

    C. Knight Aldrich
    Robert L. Arnstein
    Ezra Griffith
    Steve Katz
    W. Walter Menninger

---

*Deceased.

Consultants
  John C. Nemiah
  Henry H. Work

Ex-Officio
  John Schowalter
  Carolyn B. Robinowitz

CONTRIBUTORS

GAP Publications

Adolescent Suicide (GAP Report 140, 1996), Formulated by the Committee on Adolescence

Mental Health in Remote Rural Developing Areas: Concepts and Cases (GAP Report 139, 1995), Formulated by the Committee on Therapeutic Care

Introduction to Occupational Psychiatry (GAP Report 138, 1994), Formulated by the Committee on Occupational Psychiatry

Forced Into Treatment: The Role of Coercion in Clinical Practice (GAP Report 137, 1994), Formulated by the Committee on Government Policy

Resident's Guide to Treatment of People With Chronic Mental Illness (GAP Report 136, 1993), Formulated by the Committee on Psychiatry and the Community

Caring for People With Physical Impairment: The Journey Back (GAP Report 135, 1992), Formulated by the Committee on Handicaps

Beyond Symptom Suppression: Improving Long-Term Outcomes of Schizophrenia (GAP Report 134, 1992), Formulated by the Committee on Psychopathology

Psychotherapy in the Future (GAP Report 133, 1992), Formulated by the Committee on Therapy

---

*Title is out of print.
†Available from Books on Demand, University Microfilms International, 300 North Zeeb Road, Ann Arbor, MI 48106-1346 (800-521-0600, ext. 3492).

Leaders and Followers: A Psychiatric Perspective on Religious Cults (GAP Report 132, 1992), Formulated by the Committee on Psychiatry and Religion

The Mental Health Professional and the Legal System (GAP Report 131, 1991), Formulated by the Committee on Psychiatry and the Law

***Psychotherapy With College Students** (GAP Report 130, 1990), Formulated by the Committee on the College Student

A Casebook in Psychiatric Ethics (GAP Report 129, 1990), Formulated by the Committee on Medical Education

***Suicide and Ethnicity in the United States** (GAP Report 128, 1989), Formulated by the Committee on Cultural Psychiatry

Psychiatric Prevention and the Family Life Cycle: Risk Reduction by Frontline Practitioners (GAP Report 127, 1989), Formulated by the Committee on Preventive Psychiatry

How Old Is Old Enough? The Ages of Rights and Responsibilities (GAP Report 126, 1989), Formulated by the Committee on Child Psychiatry

The Psychiatric Treatment of Alzheimer's Disease (GAP Report 125, 1988), Formulated by the Committee on Aging

Speaking Out for Psychiatry: A Handbook for Involvement With the Mass Media (GAP Report 124, 1987), Formulated by the Committee on Public Education

Us and Them: The Psychology of Ethnonationalism (GAP Report 123, 1987), Formulated by the Committee on International Relations

Psychiatry and Mental Health Professionals (GAP Report 122, 1987), Formulated by the Committee on Governmental Agencies

Interactive Fit: A Guide to Nonpsychotic Chronic Patients (GAP Report 121, 1987), Formulated by the Committee on Psychopathology

Teaching Psychotherapy in Contemporary Psychiatric Residency Training (GAP Report 120, 1986), Formulated by the Committee on Therapy

A Family Affair: Helping Families Cope With Mental Illness: A Guide for the Professions (GAP Report 119, 1986), Formulated by the Committee on Psychiatry and the Community

Crises of Adolescence—Teenage Pregnancy: Impact on Adolescent Development (GAP Report 118, 1986), Formulated by the Committee on Adolescence

The Family, the Patient, and the Psychiatric Hospital: Toward a New Model (GAP Report 117, 1985), Formulated by the Committee on Family

Research and the Complex Causality of the Schizophrenias (GAP
Report 116, 1984), Formulated by the Committee on Research
*Friends and Lovers in the College Years (GAP Report 115, 1983), For-
mulated by the Committee on the College Student
*Mental Health and Aging: Approaches to Curriculum Development
(GAP Report 114, 1983), Formulated by the Committee on Aging
Community Psychiatry: A Reappraisal (GAP Report 113, 1983), For-
mulated by the Committee on Psychiatry and the Community
The Child and Television Drama (GAP Report 112, 1982), Formulated
by the Committee on Social Issues
*The Process of Child Therapy (GAP Report 111, 1982), Formulated by
the Committee on Child Psychiatry
**The Positive Aspects of Long-Term Hospitalization in the Public Sec-
tor for Chronic Psychiatric Patients** (GAP Report 110, 1982), Formulated by the Committee on Psychopathology
Job Loss—A Psychiatric Perspective (GAP Report 109, 1982), Formulated by the Committee on Psychiatry in Industry
A Survival Manual for Medical Students (GAP Report 108, 1982), For-
mulated by the Committee on Medical Education
**INTERFACES: A Communication Casebook for Mental Health Deci-
sion Makers** (GAP Report 107, 1981), Formulated by the Commit-
tee on Mental Health Services
*Divorce, Child Custody and the Family (GAP Report 106, 1980), For-
mulated by the Committee on Family
*Mental Health and Primary Medical Care (GAP Report 105, 1980),
Formulated by the Committee on Preventive Psychiatry
Psychiatric Consultation in Mental Retardation (GAP Report 104, 1979),
Formulated by the Committee on Mental Retardation
*Self-Involvement in the Middle East Conflict (GAP Report 103, 1978),
Formulated by the Committee on International Relations
The Chronic Mental Patient in the Community (GAP Report 102, 1978),
Formulated by the Committee on Psychiatry and the Community
**Power and Authority in Adolescence: The Origins and Resolutions of
Intergenerational Conflict** (GAP Report 101, 1978), Formulated by
the Committee on Adolescence
***Psychotherapy and Its Financial Feasibility Within the National
Health Care System** (GAP Report 100, 1978), Formulated by the
Committee on Therapy
*†What Price Compensation? (GAP Report 99, 1977), Formulated by
the Committee on Psychiatry in Industry

*Psychiatry and Sex Psychopath Legislation: The 30s to the 80s (GAP Report 98, 1977), Formulated by the Committee on Psychiatry and Law

Mysticism: Spiritual Quest or Psychic Disorder? (GAP Report 97, 1976), Formulated by the Committee on Psychiatry and Religion

*†Recertification: A Look at the Issues (GAP Report 96, 1976), Formulated by the Ad hoc Committee on Recertification

*†The Effect of the Method of Payment on Mental Health Care Practice (GAP Report 95, 1975), Formulated by the Committee on Governmental Agencies

*The Psychiatrist and Public Welfare Agencies (GAP Report 94, 1975), Formulated by the Committee on Psychiatry and the Community

*Pharmacotherapy and Psychotherapy: Paradoxes, Problems and Progress (GAP Report 93, 1975), Formulated by the Committee on Research

*The Educated Woman: Prospects and Problems (GAP Report 92, 1975), Formulated by the Committee on the College Student

*†The Community Worker: A Response to Human Need (GAP Report 91, 1974), Formulated by the Committee on Therapeutic Care

*†Problems of Psychiatric Leadership (GAP Report 90, 1974), Formulated by the Committee on Therapy

*Misuse of Psychiatry in the Criminal Courts: Competency to Stand Trial (GAP Report 89, 1974), Formulated by the Committee on Psychiatry and Law

Assessment of Sexual Function: A Guide to Interviewing (GAP Report 88, 1973), Formulated by the Committee on Medical Education

From Diagnosis to Treatment: An Approach to Treatment Planning for the Emoti onally Disturbed Child (GAP Report 87, 1973), Formulated by the Committee on Child Psychiatry

*†Humane Reproduction (GAP Report 86, 1973), Formulated by the Committee on Preventive Psychiatry

*The Welfare System and Mental Health (GAP Report 85, 1973), Formulated by the Committee on Psychiatry and Social Work

*†The Joys and Sorrows of Parenthood (GAP Report 84, 1973), Formulated by the Committee on Public Education

*The VIP With Psychiatric Impairment (GAP Report 83, 1973), Formulated by the Committee on Governmental Agencies

*Crisis in Child Mental Health: A Critical Assessment (GAP Report 82, 1972), Formulated by the Ad hoc Committee

The Aged and Community Mental Health: A Guide to Program Development (GAP Report 81, 1971), Formulated by the Committee on Aging

*Drug Misuse: A Psychiatric View of a Modern Dilemma** (GAP Report 80, 1970), Formulated by the Committee on Mental Health Services

*†Toward a Public Policy on Mental Health Care of the Elderly** (GAP Report 79, 1970), Formulated by the Committee on Aging

The Field of Family Therapy (GAP Report 78, 1970), Formulated by the Committee on Family

*Toward Therapeutic Care** (2nd Edition—No. 51 revised) (GAP Report 77, 1970), Formulated by the Committee on Therapeutic Care

*The Case History Method in the Study of Family Process** (GAP Report 76, 1970), Formulated by the Committee on Family

*The Right to Abortion: A Psychiatric View** (GAP Report 75, 1969), Formulated by the Committee on Psychiatry and Law

*†The Psychiatrist and Public Issues** (GAP Report 74, 1969), Formulated by the Committee on International Relations

*†Psychotherapy and the Dual Research Tradition** (GAP Report 73, 1969), Formulated by the Committee on Therapy

*Crisis in Psychiatric Hospitalization** (GAP Report 72, 1969), Formulated by the Committee on Therapeutic Care

*On Psychotherapy and Casework** (GAP Report 71, 1969), Formulated by the Committee on Psychiatry and Social Work

*The Nonpsychotic Alcoholic Patient and the Mental Hospital** (GAP Report 70, 1968), Formulated by the Committee on Mental Health Services

*The Dimensions of Community Psychiatry** (GAP Report 69, 1968), Formulated by the Committee on Preventive Psychiatry

*Normal Adolescence** (GAP Report 68, 1968), Formulated by the Committee on Adolescence

The Psychic Function of Religion in Mental Illness and Health (GAP Report 67, 1968), Formulated by the Committee on Psychiatry and Religion

*Mild Mental Retardation: A Growing Challenge to the Physician** (GAP Report 66, 1967), Formulated by the Committee on Mental Retardation

*†The Recruitment and Training of the Research Psychiatrist** (GAP Report 65, 1967), Formulated by the Committee on Psychopathology

*Education for Community Psychiatry (GAP Report 64, 1967), Formu-
    lated by the Committee on Medical Education
*†Psychiatric Research and the Assessment of Change (GAP Report
    63, 1966), Formulated by the Committee on Research
*Psychopathological Disorders in Childhood: Theoretical Consider-
    ations and a Proposed Classification (GAP Report 62, 1966), For-
    mulated by the Committee on Child Psychiatry
*Laws Governing Hospitalization of the Mentally Ill (GAP Report 61,
    1966), Formulated by the Committee on Psychiatry and Law
*Sex and the College Student (GAP Report 60, 1965), Formulated by
    the Committee on the College Student
*†Psychiatry and the Aged: An Introductory Approach (GAP Report
    59, 1965), Formulated by the Committee on Aging
*†Medical Practice and Psychiatry: The Impact of Changing Demands
    (GAP Report 58, 1964), Formulated by the Committee on Public
    Education
Psychiatric Aspects of the Prevention of Nuclear War (GAP Report 57,
    1964), Formulated by the Committee on Social Issues
*Mental Retardation: A Family Crisis—The Therapeutic Role of the
    Physician (GAP Report 56, 1963), Formulated by the Committee on
    Mental Retardation
*Public Relations: A Responsibility of the Mental Hospital Administra-
    tor (GAP Report 55, 1963), Formulated by the Committee on Hospitals
*The Preclinical Teaching of Psychiatry (GAP Report 54, 1962), Formu-
    lated by the Committee on Medical Education
*Psychiatrists as Teachers in Schools of Social Work (GAP Report 53,
    1962), Formulated by the Committee on Psychiatry and Social Work
The College Experience: A Focus for Psychiatric Research (GAP
    Report 52, 1962), Formulated by the Committee on the College
    Student
*Toward Therapeutic Care: A Guide for Those Who Work With the
    Mentally Ill (GAP Report 51, 1961), Formulated by the Committee
    on Therapeutic Care
*Problems of Estimating Changes in Frequency of Mental Disorders
    (GAP Report 50, 1961), Formulated by the Committee on Preven-
    tive Psychiatry
*Reports in Psychotherapy: Initial Interviews (GAP Report 49, 1961),
    Formulated by the Committee on Therapy
*Psychiatry and Religion: Some Steps Toward Mutual Understanding
    and Usefulness (GAP Report 48, 1960), Formulated by the Com-
    mittee on Psychiatry and Religion

*Preventive Psychiatry in the Armed Forces: With Some Implications for Civilian Use (GAP Report 47, 1960), Formulated by the Committee on Governmental Agencies

*Administration of the Public Psychiatric Hospital (GAP Report 46, 1960), Formulated by the Committee on Hospitals

*Confidentiality and Privileged Communication in the Practice of Psychiatry (GAP Report 45, 1960), Formulated by the Committee on Psychiatry and Law

*The Psychiatrist and His Roles in a Mental Health Association (GAP Report 44, 1960), Formulated by the Committee on Public Education

*Basic Considerations in Mental Retardation: A Preliminary Report (GAP Report 43, 1959), Formulated by the Committee on Mental Retardation

*Some Observations on Controls in Psychiatric Research (GAP Report 42, 1959), Formulated by the Committee on Research

*Working Abroad: A Discussion of Psychological Attitudes and Adaptation in New Situations (GAP Report 41, 1958), Formulated by the Committee on International Relations

*Small Group Teaching in Psychiatry for Medical Students (GAP Report 40, 1958), Formulated by the Committee on Medical Education

*The Psychiatrist's Interest in Leisure-Time Activities (GAP Report 39, 1958), Formulated by the Committee on Public Education

The Diagnostic Process in Child Psychiatry (GAP Report 38, 1958), Formulated by the Committee on Child Psychiatry

*Emotional Aspects of School Desegregation (an abbreviated and less technical version of Report No. 37) (GAP Report 37A, 1960), Formulated by the Committee on Social Issues

*Psychiatric Aspects of School Desegregation (GAP Report 37, 1957), Formulated by the Committee on Social Issues

*The Person With Epilepsy at Work (GAP Report 36, 1957), Formulated by the Committee on Psychiatry in Industry

*The Psychiatrist in Mental Health Education: Suggestions on Collaboration With Teachers (GAP Report 35, 1956), Formulated by the Committee on Public Education

*The Consultant Psychiatrist in a Family Service Agency (GAP Report 34, 1956), Formulated by the Committee on Psychiatry and Social Work

*Therapeutic Use of the Self (A Concept for Teaching Patient Care) (GAP Report 33, 1955), Formulated by the Committee on Psychiatric Nursing

*Considerations on Personality Development in College Students (GAP Report 32, 1955), Formulated by the Committee on the College Student

*Trends and Issues in Psychiatric Residency Programs (GAP Report 31, 1955), Formulated by the Committee on Medical Education

*Report on Homosexuality With Particular Emphasis on This Problem in Governmental Agencies (GAP Report 30, 1955), Formulated by the Committee on Governmental Agencies

*The Psychiatrist in Mental Health Education (GAP Report 29, 1954), Formulated by the Committee on Public Education

*The Use of Psychiatrists in Government in Relation to International Problems (GAP Report 28, 1954), Formulated by the Committee on International Relations

*Integration and Conflict in Family Behavior (Reissued in 1968 as No. 27A) (GAP Report 27, 1954), Formulated by the Committee on Family

*Criminal Responsibility and Psychiatric Expert Testimony (GAP Report 26, 1954), Formulated by the Committee on Psychiatry and Law

*Collaborative Research in Psychopathology (GAP Report 25, 1954), Formulated by the Committee on Psychopathology

*Control and Treatment of Tuberculosis in Mental Hospitals (GAP Report 24, 1954), Formulated by the Committee on Hospitals

*Outline to Be Used as a Guide to the Evaluation of Treatment in a Public Psychiatric Hospital (GAP Report 23, 1953), Formulated by the Committee on Hospitals

*The Psychiatric Nurse in the Mental Hospital (GAP Report 22, 1952), Formulated by the Committee on Psychiatric Nursing—Committee on Hospitals

*The Contribution of Child Psychiatry to Pediatric Training and Practice (GAP Report 21, 1952), Formulated by the Committee on Child Psychiatry

*The Application of Psychiatry to Industry (GAP Report 20, 1951), Formulated by the Committee on Psychiatry in Industry

*Introduction to the Psychiatric Aspects of Civil Defense (GAP Report 19, 1951), Formulated by the Committee on Governmental Agencies

*Promotion of Mental Health in the Primary and Secondary Schools: An Evaluation of Four Projects (GAP Report 18, 1951), Formulated by the Committee on Preventive Psychiatry

*The Role of Psychiatrists in Colleges and Universities (GAP Report 17, 1951), Formulated by the Committee on Academic Education

*Psychiatric Social Work in the Psychiatric Clinic (GAP Report 16, 1950), Formulated by the Committee on Psychiatry and Social Work

*Revised Electro-Shock Therapy Report (GAP Report 15, 1950), Formulated by the Committee on Therapy

*The Problem of the Aged Patient in the Public Psychiatric Hospital (GAP Report 14, 1950), Formulated by the Committee on Hospitals

*The Social Responsibility of Psychiatry: A Statement of Orientation (GAP Report 13, 1950), Formulated by the Committee on Social Issues

*Basic Concepts in Child Psychiatry (GAP Report 12, 1950), Formulated by the Committee on Child Psychiatry

*The Position of Psychiatrists in the Field of International Relations (GAP Report 11, 1950), Formulated by the Committee on International Relations

*Psychiatrically Deviated Sex Offenders (GAP Report 10, 1950), Formulated by the Committee on Forensic Psychiatry

*The Relation of Clinical Psychology to Psychiatry (GAP Report 9, 1949), Formulated by the Committee on Clinical Psychology

*An Outline for Evaluation of a Community Program in Mental Hygiene (GAP Report 8, 1949), Formulated by the Committee on Cooperation With Lay Groups

*Statistics Pertinent to Psychiatry in the United States (GAP Report 7, 1949), Formulated by the Committee on Hospitals

*Research on Prefrontal Lobotomy (GAP Report 6, 1948), Formulated by the Committee on Research

*Public Psychiatric Hospitals (GAP Report 5, 1948), Formulated by the Committee on Hospitals

*Commitment Procedures (GAP Report 4, 1948), Formulated by the Committee on Forensic Psychiatry

*Report on Medical Education (GAP Report 3, 1948), Formulated by the Committee on Medical Education

*The Psychiatric Social Worker in the Psychiatric Hospital (GAP Report 2, 1948), Formulated by the Committee on Psychiatric Social Work

*Shock Therapy (GAP Report 1, 1947), Formulated by the Committee on Therapy

Index to GAP Publications #1–#80

Symposia Reports

The Right to Die: Decision and Decision Makers (S-12, 1973), Formulated by the Committee on Aging

*****Death and Dying: Attitudes of Patient and Doctor** (S-11, 1965), Formulated by the Committee on Aging

*****Urban America and the Planning of Mental Health Services** (S-10, 1964), Formulated by the Committee on Preventive Psychiatry

*****Pavlovian Conditioning and American Psychiatry** (S-9, 1964), Formulated by the Committee on Research

*****Medical Uses of Hypnosis** (S-8, 1962), Formulated by the Committee on Medical Education

*****Application of Psychiatric Insights to Cross-Cultural Communication** (S-7, 1961), Formulated by the Committee on International Relations

*****The Psychological and Medical Aspects of the Use of Nuclear Energy** (S-6, 1960), Formulated by the Committee on Social Issues

*****Some Considerations of Early Attempts in Cooperation Between Religion and Psychiatry** (S-5, 1958), Formulated by the Committee on Psychiatry and Religion

*****Methods of Forceful Indoctrination: Observations and Interviews** (S-4, 1957), Formulated by the Committee on Social Issues

*****Factors Used to Increase the Susceptibility of Individuals to Forceful Indoctrination: Observations and Experiment** (S-3, 1956), Formulated by the Committee on Social Issues

*****Illustrative Strategies for Research in Psychopathology in Mental Health** (S-2, 1956), Formulated by the Committee on Psychopathology

*****Considerations Regarding the Loyalty Oath as a Manifestation of Current Social Tension and Anxiety** (S-1, 1954), Formulated by the Committee on Social Issues

Films

*****Discussion Guide to the Film** (2, 1970)
*****A Nice Kid Like You** (1, 1970)

Index

DATE DUE